Understanding Hair Loss in Men

Causes, Solutions, and Treatments

CRAFTED BY SKRIUWER

Copyright © 2024 by Skriuwer.

All rights reserved. No part of this book may be used or reproduced in any form whatsoever without written permission except in the case of brief quotations in critical articles or reviews.

For more information, contact : **kontakt@skriuwer.com** (www.skriuwer.com)

TABLE OF CONTENTS

CHAPTER 1: INTRODUCTION TO HAIR LOSS IN MEN

- Looks at how common hair loss is and why it matters
- Explores early signs, myths, and general concerns
- Highlights the range of causes, from genetics to lifestyle

CHAPTER 2: HOW HAIR GROWS AND WHY IT MATTERS

- Outlines the phases of the hair growth cycle
- Describes the structure of hair and follicles
- Explains factors that can disrupt normal growth

CHAPTER 3: ANDROGENETIC ALOPECIA EXPLAINED

- Defines the most common form of male hair loss
- Explores the hormonal link, especially with DHT
- Reviews medical and lifestyle approaches for this condition

CHAPTER 4: OTHER TYPES OF MALE HAIR LOSS

- Discusses less typical causes like alopecia areata and telogen effluvium
- Covers scarring and traction alopecia
- Explains diagnostic methods for uncommon patterns

CHAPTER 5: HORMONES AND THEIR EFFECTS ON HAIR

- Focuses on the endocrine system's role in hair
- Looks at thyroid, cortisol, and other hormones beyond DHT
- Discusses testing and balancing hormone levels

CHAPTER 6: GENETICS AND FAMILY HISTORY

- Explains how genetic traits affect follicle sensitivity
- Covers inheritance patterns and misconceptions
- Addresses testing options, including genetic markers

CHAPTER 7: LIFESTYLE CHOICES & THEIR INFLUENCE

- Examines how diet, stress, and habits can worsen or ease hair loss
- Considers smoking and alcohol impacts
- Highlights ways to modify daily routines to support hair health

CHAPTER 8: THE TRICHOTEST

- Describes what the TrichoTest is and how it works
- Outlines who might benefit from genetic insights
- Discusses applying the test results to treatment decisions

CHAPTER 9: NON-MEDICAL TIPS FOR MANAGING HAIR LOSS

- Suggests styling methods and gentle hair care techniques
- Advises on scalp massages, oils, and minimal routines
- Covers emotional support tactics without medications

CHAPTER 10: MEDICAL TREATMENTS & MEDICATIONS

- Surveys finasteride, minoxidil, and similar options
- Details how each medication works and potential side effects
- Suggests combining medical therapies with lifestyle changes

CHAPTER 11: HAIR CARE METHODS FOR HEALTHIER STRANDS

- Explores shampoos, conditioners, and other products
- Advises on washing frequency and avoiding breakage
- Recommends routines for various hair types and scalp conditions

CHAPTER 12: SURGICAL PROCEDURES AND THEIR OUTCOMES

- Discusses hair transplants (FUT vs. FUE)
- Reviews preparation, recovery, and post-op care
- Considers scalp micropigmentation and other surgical alternatives

CHAPTER 13: FUTURE TRENDS IN HAIR LOSS SOLUTIONS

- Looks at emerging research like hair cloning and gene therapy
- Covers advancements in laser devices and stem cell approaches
- Examines potential benefits and ethical considerations

CHAPTER 14: IMPORTANT NUTRIENTS AND DIETARY FACTORS

- Covers vitamins, minerals, and proteins essential for hair
- Explains the impact of deficiencies on shedding
- Suggests balanced eating plans and realistic supplement use

CHAPTER 15: EMOTIONAL IMPACT AND WAYS TO COPE

- Focuses on self-esteem issues tied to hair loss
- Discusses coping strategies and stress management
- Highlights counseling, support groups, and mindset shifts

CHAPTER 16: DEBUNKING COMMON MYTHS

- Clears up misunderstandings about hats, shampoos, or styling
- Explains genetic realities and hormone misconceptions
- Encourages fact-checking and professional guidance

CHAPTER 17: BUILDING A SUPPORT NETWORK

- Describes the benefits of family, friends, and group support
- Explains online forums, local groups, and professional counseling
- Highlights how sharing experiences fosters emotional relief

CHAPTER 18: TOOLS &TECHNOLOGY FOR HAIR LOSS

- Reviews laser caps, scalp analyzers, and tracking apps
- Explores clinical devices like robotic transplants and PRP kits
- Advises on selecting evidence-based solutions

CHAPTER 19: PERSONALIZED TREATMENT PLANS

- Stresses the need to tailor methods for each individual
- Shows how to blend medications, lifestyle changes, and support
- Suggests regular follow-ups and flexible goal-setting

CHAPTER 20: LONG-TERM MAINTENANCE AND MONITORING

- Emphasizes the ongoing nature of hair loss management
- Covers consistent checkups, adjusting therapies, and spotting relapses
- Highlights how to sustain emotional well-being and scalp health over time

Chapter 1: Introduction to Hair Loss in Men

Hair loss in men is a common event that affects millions of people across the globe. It can happen at various ages and for different reasons. Some men notice the first signs of thinning or a receding hairline while still in their early twenties. Others may not see any changes until their forties or even later. While many people think hair loss is a simple issue, it can actually be linked to many factors. These may include genes, hormone imbalances, health conditions, and habits.

In this introduction, we will look at the broad picture of male hair loss. We will note how common it is, the different ways it can look, and the basic reasons it occurs. We will also outline the parts of the scalp and hair. This will set the stage for more detailed chapters that follow.

1.1 Why Hair Loss Matters

Hair often has a social and personal meaning. It is part of a person's physical image and can affect how they view themselves. When hair begins to thin or fall out, some men feel worried or lose confidence. Changes in hair can also cause stress or a sense of vulnerability. Others might shrug it off and not pay it much mind. Both reactions are normal.

However, hair loss can be more than a cosmetic problem. Hair helps protect the scalp from sunlight and helps to regulate some aspects of temperature. A thinner scalp covering may cause sunburn more easily if proper precautions are not taken. While this might not be life-threatening, it is still an inconvenience.

1.2 A Quick Look at the Numbers

Studies show that by the age of 50, about half of men will experience some degree of pattern hair loss, also known as androgenetic alopecia. By the age of 70, this number can rise even more. But exact rates vary by region and genetic background. In some groups, there might be a higher rate of early hair loss. In others, hair thinning might occur at a slower pace.

1.3 The Many Forms of Hair Loss

Hair loss in men can appear in different shapes. The most common one is a receding hairline that starts at the temples or near the forehead. Another usual pattern is thinning at the crown, which may eventually meet the receding front, leaving a horseshoe shape around the sides of the head. Other men may experience small patches of bald spots, and in some cases, hair loss can affect the entire scalp.

1. **Androgenetic Alopecia (Male Pattern Hair Loss):** This form is largely tied to hormones and genetic factors. It often starts at the temples and crown. Over time, these thinning areas can spread if left untreated.
2. **Telogen Effluvium:** This is a form of shedding that can happen after stress on the body. Examples include major surgery, high fever, or a traumatic life event. In these cases, hair shifts more quickly into the resting stage, causing more hair to fall out at once.
3. **Alopecia Areata:** This is an autoimmune condition in which the body's immune system attacks hair follicles. The result is often round bald patches that can show up suddenly. It can progress to the entire scalp or even all body hair in some cases.
4. **Other Types:** There are various other forms, but most men will show some form of the above conditions if they notice hair thinning or bald patches.

1.4 Factors That Trigger Hair Loss

Hair loss can be triggered by many factors:

- **Genes:** Many men who lose hair have a family history of hair loss. Certain genes can make hair follicles more sensitive to a hormone called dihydrotestosterone (DHT). This results in thinner hair over time.
- **Hormones:** Shifts in hormones, such as testosterone and its byproduct DHT, can affect how hair grows or falls out.
- **Health Conditions:** Thyroid problems, infections, or chronic diseases can slow down hair growth or cause thinning.

- **Medications:** Some drugs for high blood pressure, arthritis, depression, or heart issues can lead to hair thinning as a side effect.
- **Habits and Routine:** Poor diet, smoking, or lack of rest may worsen hair loss. Overuse of harsh styling products can also weaken hair.

1.5 Early Signs of Hair Loss

Early signs of hair loss can be easy to miss. Many men do not notice a receding hairline until they compare old photos. Others might see more hair on their pillow or in the shower drain. Some notice that their hair feels thinner when running a hand through it. Another sign can be seeing more scalp when standing under bright light or in front of a mirror.

1.6 Emotional Effects

Hair loss can trigger worries about personal appearance. For some, thinning hair can cause a drop in self-esteem. These emotional effects can have a daily impact, affecting how a person might choose to style themselves or even whether they want to participate in social events. It is important to recognize that these feelings are common and that answers are available.

In future chapters, we will focus on methods that may help reduce or slow hair loss. We will also look at proven ways to manage the emotional challenges, including speaking with professionals or finding support in local groups or online forums.

1.7 The Importance of Understanding

Learning the basics about male hair loss helps individuals decide what steps to take. There is no single cause or single treatment that works for everyone. Instead, it may take testing, changes to daily routines, and visits to health experts. By having a clear view of what triggers hair loss, men can choose answers that match their personal situation.

1.8 Goals of This Book

1. **Explain Hair Growth:** We will explore how hair grows and why it sometimes stops growing.
2. **Identify Causes:** We will list the many causes of hair loss in men, including hormones, genes, and health problems.
3. **Discuss Solutions:** We will look at changes in daily habits, medical treatments, and cosmetic procedures.
4. **Long-Term Strategies:** We will look at how to maintain healthy hair once improvements have been made.
5. **Practical Tips:** We will provide tips that can be done at home to support hair health.

1.9 A Glimpse at Future Chapters

Upcoming chapters will cover detailed explanations of the hair growth cycle. We will also explain the role of hormones like testosterone. There will be a chapter on genetics and how they shape the likelihood of hair loss. Another chapter will look at how daily routines such as diet, physical activity, and stress can affect the scalp. We will also feature a section on advanced tests, like the TrichoTest, which can help reveal a person's genetic markers.

In addition, we will cover both non-medical methods (like the use of mild shampoos, scalp massage techniques, and certain hairstyles that reduce pulling) and medical solutions (like finasteride or minoxidil) in later parts of the book. We will also look at surgical options, such as hair transplants, and weigh the pros and cons.

1.10 Key Points to Remember

1. **Hair loss is Common:** Many men face thinning hair at some point.
2. **Multiple Causes:** There can be many reasons, including heredity, hormones, and lifestyle.
3. **Different Forms:** Not all hair loss looks the same. Recognizing the pattern helps in finding a fix.
4. **Impact on Daily Life:** It can affect self-image, but there are ways to cope.

5. **Knowledge is Power:** Understanding hair loss is the best way to manage it.

1.11 Honest Approach

It is important to avoid promises that sound too good to be true. While there are many techniques and solutions for hair loss, results can vary. Some men may find success with certain treatments, while others need a more thorough approach. The best path often involves a visit to a specialist and ongoing upkeep.

1.12 Looking Ahead

The next chapter will cover the structure of hair itself, explaining how it grows and the phases it passes through. This is vital to understanding what causes hair thinning. With each chapter, readers will gain a better sense of what is possible and what steps to consider.

Chapter 2: How Hair Grows and Why It Matters

Understanding how hair grows is an important step for anyone looking to address hair loss. The human hair growth cycle has distinct phases that each hair strand goes through. These phases include growing, transitioning, resting, and shedding. If there is a disruption in any of these stages, it can result in hair loss or thinning.

This chapter will explore the structure of the hair shaft, the stages of hair growth, and the reasons these stages may be disrupted. We will also discuss how scalp health and daily routines can keep these growth phases balanced.

2.1 Basic Structure of Hair

Each strand of hair consists of three main parts:

1. **Cuticle:** This is the thin outer layer that protects the internal parts of the hair. It looks like overlapping scales under a microscope. When the cuticle is smooth, hair appears shiny and resists damage better.
2. **Cortex:** This is the middle layer that makes up the bulk of the hair's structure. It contains the protein keratin, which gives hair strength, and it also holds the pigment (melanin) that gives hair its color.
3. **Medulla:** This is the innermost layer of the hair strand. It is not always present in fine hair. In thicker hair, it can play a role in giving the strand its thickness or shape.

Beneath the skin, there is the hair follicle. The follicle is a tiny organ in the scalp where hair develops. At the base of the follicle is the hair bulb, which houses cells that divide to form the hair shaft. Blood vessels in the scalp provide nutrients to these cells, supporting hair growth.

2.2 The Hair Growth Cycle

There are four main phases in the hair growth cycle. Each strand is in a different phase at any given time.

1. **Anagen (Growth Phase):** This is the longest phase. Hair strands can stay in this stage for two to six years, or even longer for some individuals. During anagen, cells in the hair bulb divide, and the hair grows at a rate of about 0.3 millimeters per day on average.
2. **Catagen (Transition Phase):** This phase lasts for about two to three weeks. The hair follicle shrinks, and the strand separates from the blood supply. This means the hair no longer grows actively.
3. **Telogen (Resting Phase):** During this stage, the hair follicle is at rest. It usually lasts for about three months. The hair strand remains in place but is not growing.
4. **Exogen (Shedding Phase):** This is sometimes considered part of the telogen phase, but many experts list it separately. During exogen, the old hair falls out. A new hair may begin growing in the follicle, returning to the anagen phase.

Under normal conditions, about 85–90% of scalp hairs are in the anagen phase, with the remaining in catagen, telogen, or exogen. Each day, a person might shed around 50–100 hairs. This is considered typical. When there is a shift in the ratio of hairs in each phase—such as a greater number of hairs in telogen or exogen than usual—a person may see more hair on their pillow or in their brush.

2.3 Factors That Can Disrupt the Growth Cycle

1. **Hormones:** A change in hormones—like an increase in dihydrotestosterone (DHT)—can cause more hair follicles to enter a shorter growth phase.
2. **Stress:** High stress can push more hairs into the resting or shedding phase. This is often called telogen effluvium.
3. **Medication:** Certain drugs, like some used for cancer treatment, can cause sudden hair fall during the growth phase.
4. **Health Conditions:** Illnesses, nutrient deficiencies, and autoimmune problems can interfere with normal growth patterns.

5. **Physical Damage:** Rough brushing, harsh chemicals, or tight hairstyles can damage the cuticle and disrupt the hair shaft structure.

2.4 The Scalp's Role

The scalp is the environment in which hair grows. If the scalp is not healthy, hair follicles can be harmed. Conditions like eczema, psoriasis, or fungal infections can block the follicle or cause inflammation, leading to hair thinning or loss. Maintaining a clean scalp is important, but extreme methods (like washing too often with harsh products) can strip away natural oils and irritate the skin.

2.5 Key Nutrients for Healthy Hair Growth

1. **Protein:** Hair is made mostly of protein. A lack of protein in the diet can lead to weak, brittle hair.
2. **Iron:** Low iron levels can reduce the oxygen delivered to the scalp, weakening follicles.
3. **Zinc:** Helps repair hair tissue and keep the oil glands around the follicles in good shape.
4. **Vitamins:** Vitamins A, C, D, and some B vitamins (like Biotin) are known to support hair structure and scalp health.
5. **Fatty Acids:** Omega-3 fatty acids can support the scalp and help control dryness.

2.6 How Age Affects the Hair Growth Cycle

As people age, the rate of cell division in the hair follicles can slow down. The length of the anagen phase might shorten, so hair spends less time growing and may fall out sooner. Some men start to notice this in their twenties or thirties, while others see it later. This is often tied to hormonal shifts that happen over time.

2.7 Common Signs of a Disturbed Growth Cycle

1. **Excessive Shedding:** Finding clumps of hair on a pillow or in the shower drain.

2. **Slower Growth:** Hair seems to take longer to achieve a certain length.
3. **Miniaturized Hairs:** The new hairs growing in might appear thinner and weaker, especially near the hairline.
4. **Patchy Areas:** Some men see gaps or sparse regions on the scalp, which can be a sign of an uneven hair cycle.

2.8 Unusual Facts to Consider

- Some research suggests that scalp tension, caused by factors like certain headwear or muscle tightness, could play a role in certain kinds of hair thinning. While not always recognized by all doctors, some experts think reducing scalp tension might help.
- Certain types of hair loss can reflect the overall health of the body. For instance, when someone experiences chronic stress, hair may move to the shedding phase earlier. Checking for underlying triggers is important.

2.9 Checking Hair Growth Patterns

If you notice changes in your hair, you can do a simple check at home. Part your hair in different areas and use a mirror or good lighting to see if there are significant changes in thickness. Some people take photos of their hair every few months to spot changes early.

Professional checks often involve a dermatologist using a magnifying tool called a dermoscope to look at the scalp more closely. They might do a "pull test," gently pulling on small sections of hair to see how many strands come out. A small scalp biopsy can also be used, though it is less common, to look at the follicles under a microscope.

2.10 Protecting the Hair Growth Cycle

1. **Gentle Care:** Use mild shampoos, avoid extreme heat styling, and handle wet hair carefully.
2. **Healthy Scalp:** Keep the scalp clean to reduce the risk of infections or buildup. Use products made for your scalp type.

3. **Balanced Eating:** Include sources of protein, iron, and vitamins in your meals.
4. **Stress Management:** Practices such as simple breathing exercises or hobbies can help reduce stress-related hair loss.
5. **Avoid Harsh Treatments:** Be mindful about chemical treatments like bleaching or perms. They can weaken the cuticle and the cortex.

2.11 How This Links to Male Hair Loss

Male pattern baldness, or androgenetic alopecia, is closely connected with changes in the hair growth cycle. In this condition, DHT causes follicles to shrink, producing finer and shorter hairs. Over time, the growth phase may become so short that new hairs barely emerge from the scalp.

In other conditions, like alopecia areata, immune cells attack the follicles, shutting down growth. In telogen effluvium, more hairs enter the resting or shedding phase earlier than they should. So, while each condition has different triggers, they all involve disruptions to the normal growth cycle.

2.12 Making Sense of Hair Care Products

The market has many hair care products. Some promise thicker, fuller hair, while others focus on repairing damage. It can be tricky to know what actually helps. Generally, products that nourish the scalp and protect the hair cuticle are beneficial. Some shampoos contain mild ingredients with balanced pH levels. Conditioners may add a protective layer to the strands, preventing dryness.

However, if a product claims it can perform miracles overnight, it may not be reliable. Real changes to the hair growth cycle take time. Hair grows, on average, about one centimeter per month, so results from a new product usually need at least a few weeks or months to become visible.

2.13 Lifestyle Choices That Influence Hair Growth

1. **Smoking:** Studies link smoking to faster hair thinning. Chemicals in smoke can affect blood flow to the scalp.

2. **Alcohol Overuse:** Drinking too much can lead to poor nutrient absorption, hurting hair health.
3. **Poor Sleep:** Hair growth and cell repair mostly happen during sleep. Not getting enough rest can slow these processes.
4. **Exercise:** A moderate amount of exercise supports circulation, which can help hair follicles. Overtraining, though, may raise cortisol levels and lead to stress-related hair issues.

2.14 Professional Treatments That Target Growth

Aside from the basics, some clinics offer scalp treatments like low-level laser therapy. Some men find that these sessions, which use light energy to stimulate the follicles, help with mild forms of hair thinning. There are also specialized products containing minoxidil or finasteride that focus on extending the anagen phase or blocking DHT.

2.15 Innovative Observations

- Investigations in hair cloning and stem cell therapy are underway. In theory, specialists might one day be able to grow new follicles in a lab and transplant them to the scalp.
- Scientists are studying the impact of "microbiome" on the scalp, the mix of bacteria and fungi on the skin's surface. An imbalance could lead to issues like dandruff or inflammation.

2.16 When to Seek Help

If you notice large amounts of hair in the sink or on your brush and see signs of scalp irritation, it might be time to speak with a professional. Some men wait until half of their hair is gone before seeking help, which may limit the effectiveness of some solutions. Early diagnosis can make a real difference.

2.17 Guidance for Home Experiments

Some people like to try different do-it-yourself methods, such as applying natural oils like coconut oil, olive oil, or castor oil to the scalp. Although some oils can moisturize and might help protect hair from breakage, they do not always fix hair loss rooted in hormonal or genetic causes. However, a healthy scalp environment can still offer benefits.

2.18 Putting Knowledge into Practice

If you understand the normal phases of hair growth, you can watch for early warning signs. You can also adopt daily routines that keep each phase strong. For example, not skipping breakfast can ensure your body has the energy needed to support hair cells. Adding protein-rich foods may also help sustain the anagen phase.

2.19 Summary of Chapter 2

- Hair strands follow a cycle of growth, transition, rest, and shedding.
- The scalp plays a big role in maintaining healthy follicles.
- Disruptions in the growth cycle can be caused by hormones, stress, poor nutrition, or scalp problems.
- Men who experience hair loss often have a change in how long the growth phase lasts.
- Simple care steps, such as gentle washing, balanced diets, and stress control, can help protect hair.

2.20 Looking Ahead

In upcoming chapters, we will focus on specific types of hair loss that men commonly face. We will also look at how hormones and genetics make some men more likely to experience hair loss than others. Later, we will discuss advanced testing options, including the TrichoTest, which can help personalize treatment plans.

By recognizing that hair growth relies on a delicate cycle, men can better appreciate why some treatments require time and consistent effort. The next chapters will dive deeper into hormone roles, especially androgens, and how they impact the hair follicle.

Chapter 3: Androgenetic Alopecia Explained

Androgenetic alopecia, often called male pattern baldness, is the most widespread form of hair loss in men. This condition is closely tied to hormones and genetic factors. While it is common, there are still many misunderstandings about how it works and why some men see it at an early age while others may keep a full head of hair for decades.

In this chapter, we will explore the science behind androgenetic alopecia, key signals to watch for, and how experts classify various levels of thinning. We will also cover ways it can be slowed or handled, both medically and in daily life.

3.1 Basic Explanation of Androgenetic Alopecia

Androgenetic alopecia involves a strong link to a hormone byproduct called dihydrotestosterone (DHT). Testosterone, the main male hormone, is converted into DHT by an enzyme known as 5-alpha reductase. In men who have a genetic tendency for hair thinning, DHT makes certain hair follicles more prone to shrinking over time. As these follicles shrink, the hair that grows out becomes thinner and shorter.

In these sensitive follicles, the growth stage (anagen phase) becomes shorter. Hair does not have enough time to grow to its usual length and thickness before it sheds. Eventually, the follicles can close up completely. This process often follows a predictable pattern, which is why it is sometimes referred to as "pattern baldness."

3.1.1 The Role of Genes

Genes that make certain hair follicles more sensitive to DHT can come from either parent. This means a man might inherit the genes from his father's side, mother's side, or both. Even if a man's father never lost much hair, the mother's family line can carry the genes too. But not everyone with the genes will see the same level of thinning. Hormones, health conditions, and daily habits can all influence how early or severe the thinning becomes.

3.2 Signs and Stages

Androgenetic alopecia often starts with subtle changes. A man might notice his hairline receding around the temples, or a small patch of thinning at the crown. These changes might take months or even years to become apparent. The pattern is usually gradual, unlike some other conditions where patches of hair can vanish overnight.

3.2.1 Common Patterns

1. **Receding Hairline:** The hairline moves backward at the temples, forming an "M" shape.
2. **Thinning at the Crown:** A circular or oval patch of thin hair appears at the top of the head.
3. **Combination:** Both the temples and crown become thinner, eventually meeting in the middle.

3.2.2 The Norwood Scale

Doctors often use the Norwood scale (also called the Hamilton-Norwood scale) to classify the extent of male pattern baldness. It ranges from a slight recession at the temples (Stage 1 or 2) to a more advanced loss across the entire top of the head (Stage 7). This scale helps track the progress of hair loss over time and can guide treatment decisions.

3.3 Why Some Men Show It Early

Many factors decide how quickly androgenetic alopecia moves forward. Some men experience a noticeable receding hairline by their early 20s, while others might not see any change until much later. Possible reasons for early onset include:

- **Genetics:** If close relatives lost hair at a young age, there is a higher likelihood it will happen early for that person too.
- **Hormone Levels:** Higher levels of circulating testosterone or an increased amount of 5-alpha reductase enzyme can boost DHT levels.
- **Health Conditions:** Any issue that disrupts hormones, like certain thyroid conditions, may affect hair growth.
- **High Stress:** Intense stress might worsen hormonal imbalances or speed up normal thinning processes, though stress alone typically does not cause classic male pattern baldness.

3.4 Medical Approaches to Androgenetic Alopecia

Because androgenetic alopecia connects strongly with hormones and genetic makeup, medical treatments often aim to slow the impact of DHT on hair follicles. Below are some common methods that have been studied.

3.4.1 Oral Medications (5-Alpha Reductase Inhibitors)

Medications like finasteride (and in some cases dutasteride) lower the levels of DHT in the scalp by blocking the enzyme that creates it. Many men who use finasteride notice slower hair loss. Some may even see modest regrowth in thinning areas. However, the drug must be taken consistently. If a person stops, hair loss might return to what it was before.

Possible Side Effects: Some users mention reduced sex drive or mild changes in mood. These effects are not universal, but they should be discussed with a health professional before starting treatment.

3.4.2 Topical Medications

Minoxidil solution or foam can be applied directly to thinning scalp areas. It extends the anagen phase of hair growth, so more follicles remain active. This medication is typically applied twice daily. It often helps slow the rate of hair loss and can lead to some regrowth, especially in the crown area.

Key Points:

- Works best for mild to moderate cases.
- Must be used regularly to see benefits.
- Possible side effects include scalp irritation or dryness.

3.4.3 Low-Level Laser Therapy (LLLT)

Certain clinics use laser devices, such as helmets or handheld wands, that emit light energy to the scalp. The theory is that this may help improve blood flow and support healthy follicles. Studies are mixed in their conclusions, but some users report less shedding and small improvements in thickness when used regularly.

3.4.4 Platelet-Rich Plasma (PRP)

PRP involves taking a small amount of the patient's blood, separating out the growth factors, then injecting that concentration into thinning areas of the scalp. The aim is to boost the follicles' own healing process. Some individuals report improvements in hair thickness, but results can vary, and multiple sessions are often needed.

3.5 Non-Medical Methods and Routine Changes

While medical treatments directly address DHT's impact, everyday routines can also help slow or lessen visible hair loss:

1. **Gentle Styling:** Men with thinning hair might use mild styling products and avoid tight hats to reduce strain on fragile follicles.
2. **Shampoos and Conditioners:** Products designed for sensitive scalps can limit irritation, but they cannot reverse genetic hair loss alone.
3. **Nutritional Support:** While balanced nutrition may not stop androgenetic alopecia, poor eating can make thinning worse by weakening hair structure.
4. **Scalp Massage:** Some people find that gentle scalp massages with natural oils improve blood flow. They can also help relax the scalp

muscles, though scalp massage alone is not enough to reverse pattern baldness.

3.6 Misinformation and Pitfalls

Because androgenetic alopecia is so common, many products claim to cure or halt hair loss completely. One should be careful when considering new products that lack scientific support. Common pitfalls include:

- **Miracle Cures:** Some sellers promise a fast reversal of baldness, which is usually unrealistic.
- **Excessive Vitamin Use:** Overloading on supplements can cause imbalances in the body.
- **Home Remedies:** While some natural oils or extracts might provide moisture, few have shown a direct impact on DHT-driven hair loss.

3.7 Personal Factors in Treatment Choices

When deciding on a management plan, each person's situation is unique. Some men may be comfortable with mild to moderate thinning and choose not to use medications. Others may feel more motivated to try finasteride, minoxidil, or both. For advanced cases or those who do not respond to medications, surgical options like hair transplantation (discussed in a later chapter) might be an option.

It is important to consult a professional, such as a dermatologist, who can confirm that the hair loss is indeed androgenetic alopecia and not another condition. Confirming the correct diagnosis helps prevent wasting time and money on the wrong approaches.

3.8 Tips for Early Detection

Not everyone notices hair loss right away. Early detection can improve treatment outcomes, since existing follicles are easier to support than follicles that have already shrunk. A few ways to spot early problems include:

1. **Use Photographs:** Take pictures of your hairline and crown every few months under similar lighting.
2. **Watch Your Pillow or Shower Drain:** A sudden increase in shedding can signal a shift in the hair growth cycle.
3. **Feel Changes in Thickness:** Gently run your fingers through your hair in areas that seem thinner. If it feels less dense over time, it might be worth a check.

3.9 Psychological Factors

Some men become upset by the first signs of a receding hairline or thinning crown. Worries about aging, attractiveness, or social judgment can arise. These feelings are common. Talking to friends, seeking out forums, or consulting a counselor can help address negative thoughts. Approaching androgenetic alopecia with knowledge and realistic goals can reduce stress in the long run.

3.10 Innovative Observations in Research

Research in the field continues, with scientists looking into new strategies:

- **Stem Cell Studies:** Experts are exploring how to re-activate dormant hair follicles or even generate new ones.
- **Gene Therapy:** In the future, it may be possible to switch off or modify genes that make follicles prone to shrinkage.
- **Localized Inhibitors:** New treatments aim to more directly block DHT only in the scalp, reducing possible side effects seen with oral medications.

Although these ideas are still in development, they represent hopeful areas for men who want more options.

Chapter 4: Other Types of Male Hair Loss

Androgenetic alopecia is the best-known form of hair loss in men, but there are other types that can appear. These conditions may have different causes, such as stress, immune system issues, or physical damage. Each type needs a separate plan for diagnosis and management.

In this chapter, we will outline some of the most common alternative hair loss conditions, including their main signs, typical triggers, and potential treatments. This information can help men and health professionals better decide when to rule out or confirm male pattern baldness, or if something else is causing the thinning.

4.1 Telogen Effluvium

Telogen effluvium is a condition where more hair than normal enters the resting (telogen) phase and then falls out in a short period. Men with telogen effluvium often see a sudden increase in shedding. Their scalp might look noticeably thinner, but bald patches are not always present.

4.1.1 Common Triggers

- **Major Surgery:** The body focuses on healing, causing resources to shift away from hair growth.
- **High Fever or Severe Infection:** Extreme health stress can disrupt the hair cycle.
- **Intense Stress:** Emotional or physical stress might push too many hairs into telogen phase.
- **Significant Diet Changes:** Sudden shifts in eating patterns, especially if the person is not getting enough protein or nutrients.

4.1.2 Main Signs

- Increased shedding over a few weeks or months.
- General thinning across the scalp rather than specific patches.
- Loose hairs found on pillows, combs, or in the shower.

4.1.3 Recovery and Treatment

Telogen effluvium is often temporary. Once the cause is addressed—be it stress management, improved nutrition, or recovery from illness—new hair growth usually resumes. In some men, hair can take several months to return to its former thickness.

While waiting, gentle handling of the scalp, a balanced diet, and mild hair care products can help support healthier regrowth. Sometimes, short-term use of topical solutions like minoxidil might be suggested to encourage new growth, although the results vary.

4.2 Alopecia Areata

Alopecia areata is an autoimmune condition where the body's defense system mistakenly attacks hair follicles. This leads to round or oval spots of hair loss. These patches may show up overnight in some cases. It can affect the scalp and sometimes even facial hair like beards.

4.2.1 Autoimmune Involvement

Scientists believe cells from the immune system target hair follicles, causing them to stop growing. This is different from androgenetic alopecia, which involves hormones. Alopecia areata sometimes happens alongside other autoimmune problems (for instance, thyroid issues), but not always.

4.2.2 Patchy Appearance

Unlike male pattern baldness, which follows a predictable receding pattern, alopecia areata creates random patches of hair loss. These patches can vary in size, from small coin-like areas to larger sections. In some people, the condition can progress to total hair loss on the scalp (alopecia totalis) or even the entire body (alopecia universalis).

4.2.3 Possible Treatments

- **Steroid Injections:** A doctor might inject steroids into the patches to calm the immune reaction.

- **Topical Therapies:** Steroid creams or other immune-modulating agents can sometimes help.
- **Light Therapy:** Some clinics use controlled ultraviolet light on the scalp to slow down immune attacks.
- **Minoxidil:** May be combined with other treatments to encourage new hair growth.

Recovery can happen spontaneously, with hair growing back without intervention. But it may also come and go over time, especially if the autoimmune triggers remain.

4.3 Traction Alopecia

Traction alopecia is caused by chronic pulling on the hair follicles. This can happen from wearing tight hairstyles (like tight braids) or headgear that pulls or rubs the scalp in specific areas.

4.3.1 Who Is at Risk?

Men who wear certain hats or helmets for work or sports, or who style their hair in a way that pulls on the scalp, might develop traction alopecia. The constant tension can weaken the hair shaft and damage follicles.

4.3.2 Prevention

The simplest way to prevent traction alopecia is to avoid tight hairstyles or loosen helmets or hats that press firmly on specific areas of the scalp. Regular breaks from these stressors can help. If caught early, follicles can recover and grow hair normally. However, in severe cases where the damage is long-term, hair transplant or other interventions might be needed.

4.4 Scarring Alopecia (Cicatricial Alopecia)

Scarring alopecia involves a group of conditions where hair follicles are destroyed and replaced with scar tissue. Once a follicle has formed scar tissue, new hair usually cannot grow there. These conditions can result from infections, burns, inflammatory skin problems, or certain autoimmune disorders.

4.4.1 Examples of Scarring Conditions

- **Lichen Planopilaris:** An inflammatory scalp disorder that can lead to permanent bald spots.
- **Frontal Fibrosing Alopecia:** Causes a slow-moving band of hair loss near the front of the scalp.
- **Fungal Infections:** If severe and left untreated, they may damage follicles enough to cause scarring.

4.4.2 Management

Early detection is key. Once the follicles have scarred, the area may not recover hair growth. A doctor may do a biopsy of the scalp to confirm the diagnosis. Treatments can include anti-inflammatory drugs, antibiotics (if an infection is involved), or other prescriptions to reduce immune system attacks.

4.5 Tinea Capitis (Fungal Infection)

Tinea capitis is a fungal infection that can appear on the scalp. Children get it more often than adults, but men can still be affected. The fungus attacks the hair shafts, leading to patchy hair loss, scaling, and sometimes itching or redness. Hairs might break off at the scalp, giving the area a stubbly look.

4.5.1 Signs of Tinea Capitis

- Round patches of scaly skin on the scalp.
- Brittle hair that snaps off easily.
- Itching or slight pain in affected areas.
- Swollen glands in the neck in some cases.

4.5.2 Treatment

An oral antifungal medication is often necessary, as topical treatments alone may not penetrate deeply enough into the hair follicles. It can take several weeks or months to clear the infection. During this time, keeping the scalp clean and following a doctor's instructions are crucial.

4.6 Hair Shaft Problems

Sometimes, the hair shaft itself is fragile or malformed. Conditions like trichorrhexis nodosa involve weak points along the shaft that break easily. While this does not always result in total bald patches, the hair can appear thin or unkempt.

4.6.1 Causes of Shaft Damage

- **Excessive Heat:** Overuse of flat irons or curling devices can weaken the strand.
- **Chemical Treatments:** Repeated bleaching or coloring can strip away protective layers.
- **Physical Trauma:** Rough brushing, towel-drying, or twisting hair can create splits.

4.6.2 Improving Shaft Health

Limiting exposure to damaging practices, using gentle products, and avoiding harsh chemicals can give the hair shaft a better chance to grow normally. While this will not fix genetic or hormonal causes of thinning, it can reduce breakage and help hair look fuller.

4.7 Stress-Related Shedding and Trichotillomania

There are cases where stress plays a large part in hair loss. While stress alone may not typically cause classic bald spots, it can worsen existing conditions or contribute to temporary shedding.

4.7.1 Stress-Related Shedding

Chronic stress can push more hairs into the resting phase, similar to telogen effluvium. Reducing stress through simple relaxation methods, regular breaks, and medical advice can lead to an improvement in growth over time.

4.7.2 Trichotillomania

Trichotillomania is a condition where a person feels an urge to pull out their own hair. This is often tied to emotional or mental stress. Small or large patches of missing hair can appear, sometimes in easy-to-reach areas like the front or sides of the scalp. Therapy, counseling, or habit-reversal strategies can help manage this behavior.

4.8 Key Differences Between Various Types

Men dealing with hair loss should remember that not all thinning is male pattern baldness. Some distinctions to keep in mind:

1. **Pattern vs. Patches:** Androgenetic alopecia follows a predictable shape, while alopecia areata tends to create round patches.
2. **Speed of Loss:** Telogen effluvium can occur quickly, while androgenetic alopecia is more gradual.
3. **Pain or Itching:** Conditions involving inflammation or infection might cause discomfort, whereas male pattern baldness is usually painless.
4. **Recovery Potential:** Telogen effluvium and traction alopecia can be reversed if caught early. Scarring alopecia often leads to permanent loss.

4.9 Seeking Proper Diagnosis

When a man notices unusual or rapid hair thinning, it is wise to consult a dermatologist. A professional evaluation might include:

- **Clinical Exam:** A close look at the scalp and hair pattern.
- **Pull Test:** Checking how many hairs come out with gentle pulling.
- **Blood Tests:** Assessing hormone levels, iron levels, or possible thyroid problems.
- **Scalp Biopsy:** In more complex cases, a small piece of scalp is studied under a microscope.

Getting the right diagnosis ensures any underlying medical condition is addressed. If the cause is linked to hormones, experts can confirm whether it is indeed androgenetic alopecia or something else.

4.10 Treatment Approaches for Less Common Types

1. **Anti-Inflammatory Medicines:** Often used for autoimmune or scarring conditions.
2. **Antifungals:** Crucial for fungal infections like tinea capitis.
3. **Steroid Injections:** May help restart growth in small patches of alopecia areata.
4. **Lifestyle Adjustments:** Lessening tight hairstyles or reducing stress can be key for traction alopecia or stress shedding.
5. **Therapy for Pulling Hair:** Behavioral techniques might help those dealing with trichotillomania.

4.11 Myths Around Alternative Hair Loss

- **Myth:** All hair loss is genetic.
    - **Fact:** Many conditions, such as infections or stress-related shedding, are not linked to the genes.
- **Myth:** Applying special oils fixes bald patches instantly.
    - **Fact:** Some oils can help condition the scalp, but they do not typically cure medical problems.
- **Myth:** Wearing a hat always makes you go bald.
    - **Fact:** Normal hat-wearing does not cause permanent hair loss, though very tight hats can lead to traction alopecia if worn all the time.

4.12 Rare Causes of Hair Loss

Though not common, certain issues can also lead to thinning:

- **Nutrient Deficiencies:** Severe vitamin or mineral deficits, such as extreme low levels of zinc or protein, can harm hair.
- **Heavy Metal Poisoning:** Exposure to toxins like arsenic or thallium can lead to sudden shedding.
- **Chronic Illnesses:** Long-term diseases, including advanced stages of cancer or kidney failure, might impact the hair cycle.

In these cases, treating the main health problem or removing exposure to harmful substances is the top priority.

4.13 How Men Can Take Action

No matter the type, a few steps can help men manage or prevent further damage:

1. **Be Observant:** Watch for unusual shedding patterns or scalp changes (scales, redness, or intense itching).
2. **Seek Help Early:** A professional diagnosis can narrow down the cause and speed up treatment.
3. **Treat the Root Cause:** If hair loss is due to a fungus, for example, antifungal treatment is more important than hair growth products.
4. **Maintain Good Habits:** Adequate sleep, balanced eating, and stress reduction can support the body's natural healing.

4.14 Potential Overlaps

Men with underlying genetic hair loss might also experience telogen effluvium or traction alopecia. This can complicate the picture. A person could have a receding hairline from androgenetic alopecia while also seeing excessive shedding from emotional stress or medication side effects. That is why it is critical not to assume only one cause is at work.

4.15 Psychological Effects of Non-Pattern Hair Loss

Much like androgenetic alopecia, other forms of hair loss can lead to worry or decreased confidence. Men might feel self-conscious about patchy spots or obvious thinning. Seeking help from mental health experts or support groups can be beneficial. Knowledge about what triggers the hair loss can also reduce anxiety.

4.16 Common Treatments vs. Lesser-Known Approaches

Some men try alternative treatments like acupuncture or herbal supplements. While certain methods might improve circulation or reduce stress, their direct effect on hair regrowth is less understood. It is best to combine any alternative approach with proven medical advice for more reliable outcomes.

4.17 Practical Measures to Support Healthy Hair

- **Scalp Hygiene:** Washing with a mild shampoo keeps the scalp clean. This is especially important if scalp infections are a risk.
- **Avoid Scratching:** Persistent itching can damage follicles, especially in conditions like tinea capitis or alopecia areata.
- **Regular Checkups:** If you have a history of autoimmune problems, keep an eye on any new or recurring scalp patches.
- **Address Underlying Issues:** Whether it is stress, a fungal infection, or poor diet, the scalp's health relies on the body's overall condition.

Chapter 5: Hormones and Their Effects on Hair

Hormones play a major part in many processes in the human body. From growth and energy to mood and metabolism, these chemical messengers act as signals that tell cells and organs what to do. Hair growth is also controlled by hormones, and changes in hormone levels can be a main reason for hair thinning or baldness. In men, we often hear about testosterone and its byproduct, dihydrotestosterone (DHT), as major influences on hair. But there are other hormones that also have an impact on hair and scalp health.

In this chapter, we will explain the key hormones that affect male hair growth, how they interact with hair follicles, and what can happen when these hormones are out of balance. We will also look at how certain illnesses or medicine-related changes can alter hormone levels, causing shedding or slow regrowth. By understanding these points, men can make more informed decisions about treatment and everyday habits that might keep their hormones in check.

5.1 Basics of the Endocrine System

The endocrine system is made up of glands that produce and release hormones. These glands include the pituitary, thyroid, adrenal glands, and others. Each hormone produced has a role, and many of these roles overlap or affect other parts of the body. For example, the thyroid gland releases hormones that regulate metabolism, but thyroid imbalances can also affect hair growth and texture.

In men, the testes are a key part of the endocrine system. They produce testosterone, which is vital for male features such as facial hair and deeper voice. When testosterone enters the bloodstream, some of it is converted to DHT by an enzyme known as 5-alpha reductase. This DHT can have a powerful effect on hair follicles, especially those genetically prone to male pattern baldness.

5.2 Testosterone and Hair

Testosterone is often called the primary male hormone. It helps develop features like muscle mass and body hair. However, testosterone itself does not directly cause classic male pattern hair loss (androgenetic alopecia). The main issue is what happens when testosterone is converted into DHT.

5.2.1 Role of Testosterone in the Body

- It aids in muscle and bone strength.
- It supports sperm production in the testes.
- It influences mood and energy levels.
- It helps with body hair growth in general (face, chest, etc.).

A healthy balance of testosterone is needed for normal male health. Low levels of testosterone could lead to reduced muscle mass, fatigue, and sometimes changes in mood. On the other hand, high levels of testosterone do not always mean more scalp hair growth; in fact, too much DHT in the scalp can speed up follicle shrinking for those prone to it.

5.3 Dihydrotestosterone (DHT)

DHT is a potent hormone formed from testosterone. It binds to receptors in hair follicles, especially those in the front and top regions of the scalp in men with genetic susceptibility. Over time, DHT makes these follicles shrink. The hair that grows out becomes thinner and shorter. Eventually, the follicles may close and stop producing visible strands.

5.3.1 Why Some Follicles Are Sensitive

Not all hair follicles react the same way to DHT. For instance, hair on the sides and back of the head often remains thick even in men who are mostly bald on top. That is why hair transplant procedures often take donor hair from those "safe" zones and move them to thinning areas.

A person's genes control how sensitive certain follicles are to DHT. Men with more sensitivity might experience hair thinning earlier or at a faster rate. Others with lower sensitivity might keep a decent amount of hair longer, even if they have similar hormone levels.

5.3.2 Controlling DHT

Several medications aim to either block the enzyme 5-alpha reductase (thus reducing DHT formation) or prevent DHT from latching onto hair follicles. The most common example is finasteride, which reduces DHT levels in the scalp by blocking the enzyme. Many men who use finasteride notice less shedding and, in some cases, some regrowth.

However, blocking DHT can have other consequences, like changes in libido or mild mood effects, although not everyone experiences these. It is also important to remember that when you stop using these treatments, the protective effect is lost, and hair thinning might resume.

5.4 Other Hormones That Affect Hair

While DHT usually gets the most attention, other hormones can also have a big effect on scalp and hair.

5.4.1 Thyroid Hormones

The thyroid gland, located in the neck, produces hormones that regulate metabolism (how your body uses energy). If the thyroid is underactive (hypothyroidism) or overactive (hyperthyroidism), hair growth may slow or hair may become brittle and fall out. Men with thyroid issues might see hair changes before getting diagnosed.

1. **Hypothyroidism:** Hair may look dry or coarse, and thinning can occur across the scalp.
2. **Hyperthyroidism:** Shedding might speed up, causing a more rapid change in thickness.

Balancing thyroid hormone levels, usually through medication, often improves hair quality over time. Doctors might do a blood test to check T3, T4, and TSH (thyroid-stimulating hormone) levels if they suspect an issue.

5.4.2 Cortisol

Cortisol is often called the "stress hormone." When a person experiences high stress for a long time, cortisol levels can remain elevated. This can push more hairs into the resting phase (telogen) or cause an imbalance that leads to excessive shedding (telogen effluvium).

Chronic stress can also disrupt other hormones, adding more triggers for hair loss. While cortisol alone may not cause classic male pattern baldness, it can worsen existing issues or speed up thinning that is already underway.

5.4.3 Insulin and Blood Sugar

Insulin is the hormone that manages blood sugar. Men with insulin resistance (a sign of pre-diabetes or type 2 diabetes) might have more metabolic problems, which can also affect hair growth. Some research suggests that poor control of blood sugar can impact circulation and nutrient delivery to hair follicles.

Making sure that blood sugar is kept within normal limits can support better scalp conditions. This usually involves a balanced diet, regular physical activity, and, if needed, medical treatment for diabetes or pre-diabetes.

5.5 Life Stages and Hormonal Changes

Men experience subtle shifts in hormones through different life stages. In teenage years, testosterone levels shoot up, leading to facial hair and other traits. By the mid-20s, hormone levels are stable for many men. In the late 30s and beyond, testosterone might slowly drop each year, a process sometimes called "andropause."

Though the drop is not usually as swift as the changes that women experience in menopause, it can still be enough to affect muscle mass, mood, and possibly hair. Some men also face changes in thyroid function or other hormones as they age. Keeping track of overall health can spot problems early, allowing for timely treatment.

5.6 Hormonal Imbalances and Hair Loss

Hormonal imbalances occur if there is too much or too little of a specific hormone. This can happen because of:

1. **Gland Issues:** If a gland like the thyroid is not producing hormones properly or if there is a growth (nodule) interfering with normal function.
2. **Chronic Stress or Illness:** Long-term stress can disrupt cortisol patterns. Serious illnesses can affect multiple hormone levels.
3. **Medications:** Certain drugs for blood pressure, depression, or other conditions can shift hormone balances.
4. **Nutritional Deficiencies:** A shortage of key nutrients might reduce hormone production.

When hormones are off-balance, hair follicles may not get the right signals, leading to thinning, dryness, or slowed growth. Treating the main problem often helps hair return to a normal growth cycle.

5.7 Testing Hormone Levels

If a man shows signs of unusual or rapid hair loss, a doctor may suggest measuring hormone levels. This could include:

- **Blood Tests:** Checking testosterone, DHT, thyroid hormones, and other relevant markers (like cortisol).
- **Saliva Tests:** Sometimes used for cortisol monitoring at different times of day.

- **Urine Tests:** Rarely used but can help in special cases to measure certain hormones over a 24-hour period.

With these results, a healthcare professional can identify imbalances and suggest steps to correct them. Often, simply restoring normal thyroid or testosterone levels can improve hair health.

5.8 Medicines That Affect Hair

Some prescription drugs can disrupt hormones or the hair cycle. Common examples include:

1. **Steroids (Corticosteroids):** High doses over a long period can thin out hair.
2. **Anabolic Steroids:** Used by some athletes or bodybuilders, they can boost testosterone and DHT, triggering scalp follicle shrinking if someone is prone to it.
3. **Antidepressants:** Certain types might cause shedding in a small number of people.
4. **Blood Pressure Medicines:** Beta-blockers can sometimes affect the hair growth cycle.

If someone suspects a medication is causing thinning, it is best to speak with a doctor. Adjusting the dose or switching to another medication might ease the problem. Stopping medicine without guidance can risk other health issues, so medical advice is always important.

5.9 Balancing Hormones Through Lifestyle

Sometimes, making daily life adjustments can help keep hormones in a healthy range. While serious imbalances need medical care, mild shifts can respond well to healthier habits.

1. **Consistent Sleep:** Hormone release and regulation happen during rest. Aiming for 7-8 hours of quality sleep supports balanced hormone levels.

2. **Moderate Exercise:** Physical activity helps regulate insulin and reduces stress-related hormones. Overdoing it, however, might increase cortisol, so a balanced workout routine is key.
3. **Reduced Stress:** Relaxation methods or leisure activities can help keep cortisol under control.
4. **Nutritious Eating:** Including protein, healthy fats, and plenty of vitamins and minerals helps the body produce hormones correctly.
5. **Limit Alcohol and Smoking:** Excessive alcohol intake can disrupt testosterone, and smoking can harm circulation, including blood flow to hair follicles.

5.10 Surprising Hormone Facts

- **Interaction with Sleep:** Studies show that lack of sleep can lower testosterone levels, affecting mood and possibly hair health in the long term.
- **Gut Health Link:** There is a growing interest in how gut bacteria might influence hormone balance. A healthy digestive system may indirectly help regulate stress and other hormonal factors.
- **Seasonal Variations:** Some research suggests that testosterone and cortisol levels can shift slightly with seasons, but the impact on hair growth is usually mild.

5.11 Special Cases: Hormone Disorders

Certain rare disorders can have a direct influence on hair. For example, tumors in the pituitary gland might cause overproduction or underproduction of specific hormones. Adrenal gland disorders like Cushing's syndrome (excess cortisol) or Addison's disease (low cortisol) can change the body's overall hormone patterns and result in hair thinning or changes in texture.

If such conditions are suspected, doctors will perform imaging tests and more detailed hormone measurements to find the cause. Treatments might involve surgery, specialized medication, or a combination of both. Correcting the main disorder can often restore more normal hair growth patterns.

5.12 Myths About Hormones and Hair

- **Myth:** Bald men always have higher testosterone.
  - **Fact:** Many men with normal or even below-average testosterone can experience baldness if their follicles are very sensitive to DHT.
- **Myth:** Only male hormones matter for men's hair.
  - **Fact:** Thyroid hormones, insulin, and cortisol can also affect male hair.
- **Myth:** You can solve all hair problems with hormone replacement.
  - **Fact:** While hormone therapy might help in certain cases (like low thyroid or very low testosterone), not every hair loss case is fixed by adjusting hormones alone.

5.13 Working with a Professional

Any man concerned about hormonal causes for hair loss should consider consulting:

1. **Endocrinologist:** A doctor specializing in hormone conditions.
2. **Dermatologist:** An expert in skin and hair who can do scalp evaluations and order tests for hormone levels if needed.
3. **Primary Care Doctor:** Can identify signs of hormone-related problems and refer to a specialist if something unusual shows up in tests.

A collaborative approach can often provide the best path, since hair loss can have overlapping causes (genetics, stress, medications, etc.). Having more than one professional's input can cover all bases.

5.14 Looking Ahead: Hormone Research

Scientists continue to study the relationship between hormones and hair. Investigations look at how to precisely target hormone receptors in the scalp without affecting the rest of the body. Other studies focus on how environmental factors, such as pollution or dietary elements, might change hormone levels or their action on hair follicles.

In the future, we might see treatments that can deliver DHT blockers directly to the affected follicles, reducing overall side effects. There is also interest in gene editing tools to modify how follicles respond to hormones, though that remains experimental.

Chapter 6: Genetics and Family History

When it comes to male hair loss, one of the biggest factors is genetics. We often hear statements like, "It runs in my family," or, "My grandfather had a full head of hair, so I should be fine." There is truth to these ideas, but understanding exactly how genes affect hair follicles can be more complicated than simply looking at family pictures.

In this chapter, we will look at the science behind hereditary influences on hair. We will discuss how these genes can be passed down, why some men show signs of thinning in their twenties while others do not see changes until much later, and why the mother's side is not the only one to watch. We will also talk about other inherited traits that may affect the scalp or accelerate hair loss.

6.1 The Link Between Genes and Hair

Genes are instructions coded into DNA. They guide the body in how to develop and function. When it comes to hair, certain genes can make hair follicles more prone to the effects of hormones, like DHT. Other genes might control how quickly new hairs are produced, or how resilient they are to damage.

Men usually have half of their genes from their mother and half from their father. Both sides can contribute traits related to hair thickness, hairline shape, and how easily follicles respond to hormones. Even if one side of the family had minimal hair loss, the other side may carry strong genes for male pattern baldness.

6.2 Inheritance Patterns

The inheritance of male pattern baldness is considered "polygenic," which means multiple genes combine to shape the final outcome. It is not as simple as saying, "One gene causes baldness." Instead, each contributing gene can make a slight difference in how follicles respond to DHT or other factors.

6.2.1 The X Chromosome Myth

There is a popular myth that baldness comes only from the maternal side through the X chromosome. In reality, the picture is more diverse. While some key genes related to hair loss are indeed found on the X chromosome, there are many other genes scattered on different chromosomes that also play a part.

This is why you might see men who share a similar hair loss pattern with their father's side, their mother's side, or a mix of both. It is also why some siblings show different hair loss patterns, even though they have the same parents. The "gene shuffle" is random, making exact predictions difficult.

6.3 Early vs. Late Onset

Some men begin to see a receding hairline as early as their late teens or early twenties. Others maintain thick hair well into their thirties or beyond. Genetics can set the "clock" for when male pattern baldness starts to show. The same set of genes can also decide how rapidly thinning occurs after it begins.

For instance, if a father showed advanced thinning by 25, there is a chance his son might follow a similar pattern. But it is not guaranteed. A son's genes might not perfectly match those aspects of the father's genetic code. Environmental factors like stress, nutrition, and overall health also play a part in how quickly things move.

6.4 Types of Genetic Influence

Different genetic factors can contribute to hair structure, color, and thickness. Here are a few that might overlap with hair loss patterns:

1. **Hair Shaft Diameter Genes:** These determine how thick or thin each hair strand is. If hair is naturally thin, early thinning might be more visible.
2. **Follicle Shape and Placement:** Some genes decide how follicles are arranged on the scalp and how they grow (straight, curly, etc.).
3. **Hormone Sensitivity:** This is key in androgenetic alopecia. High sensitivity to DHT can speed up follicle shrinkage.
4. **Inflammation Tendency:** Some people are genetically prone to certain inflammatory conditions that could lead to forms of scarring alopecia or faster shedding.

6.5 Identifying Inherited Hair Loss

A good way to see if genetics play a role is to look at your closest relatives—both male and female. Do they have notable thinning, receding hairlines, or bald spots? At what age did it start? Did it progress quickly or slowly? Gathering this information can provide clues.

However, be careful: Not everyone in your family might have the same daily habits. One relative might have an active, healthy routine, while another might smoke or have poor nutrition. Environmental factors can make the same genetic tendency show up in different ways or at different times.

6.6 Genetic Testing for Hair Loss

Modern technology has made it possible to test for certain genetic markers associated with hair loss. We will discuss the TrichoTest in a dedicated chapter later, but there are other simple genetic test kits that claim to reveal a person's likelihood of future thinning. These tests look for known markers on different chromosomes linked to male pattern baldness.

6.6.1 Limits of Testing

Even if a test shows a high risk, it does not guarantee a specific outcome. Many factors, including hormones, stress, or diet, can slow or speed up genetic patterns. On the other hand, a low-risk result does not guarantee a man will keep all his hair forever. Genetic testing is only one part of the picture.

That said, knowing your genetic risk can motivate earlier action. If you learn you carry strong markers for androgenetic alopecia, you might decide to pay more attention to hair care or see a specialist at the first sign of thinning, rather than waiting until the problem is advanced.

6.7 Non-Hair-Related Genes That Can Impact Hair

Sometimes, a gene that primarily affects another part of the body can indirectly influence hair. For instance, genes tied to immune system issues might make a person more likely to develop alopecia areata. Other genes that affect hormone function (like those involving the thyroid) may cause changes in hair growth patterns.

In certain rare conditions, hair loss can be part of a larger syndrome. For example, some genetic disorders involve brittle nails and brittle hair. While not as common as androgenetic alopecia, these cases highlight that genetics can shape hair in many ways beyond just the usual pattern baldness.

6.8 Clues from Ethnic and Regional Background

Studies show that hair loss patterns can vary across populations. Some groups have a higher prevalence of early baldness, while others tend to develop it later or have it occur less frequently. This does not mean any group is immune; rather, the incidence rates differ, and that difference likely has a genetic component.

For instance, certain Mediterranean or Northern European men may have higher reported rates of androgenetic alopecia, while men from some Asian backgrounds may show a slightly lower rate. However, as populations mix, these distinctions become less clear.

6.9 Can Genes Be Altered?

One of the emerging fields in medicine is gene editing. While this is still mostly theoretical for hair loss, scientists are studying whether it is possible to block or modify genes that make hair follicles sensitive to DHT. These methods are still far from being routine, but ongoing research might open new options in the future.

Until then, men rely on treatments like finasteride, minoxidil, or hair transplantation to tackle the effects of their genetic predisposition. These methods do not change genes but aim to slow down or compensate for what the genes do to hair follicles.

6.10 The Emotional Aspect of Inherited Hair Loss

Knowing that male pattern baldness "runs in the family" can make some men feel it is inevitable. This can create stress or resignation. However, being aware of family trends can also be helpful. It gives you the chance to watch for signs earlier and take steps if needed.

Some men choose to accept their thinning hair without any problem, while others prefer to look into treatments. Both decisions are valid. The important point is that men have the information to act in a way that matches their preferences.

6.11 Tracking Family History

If you want a clearer idea of your genetic risk, you could:

1. **Ask Relatives:** Find out when they noticed changes in their hair.
2. **Examine Old Photos:** Look at pictures of relatives at different ages to see if there was a receding hairline or thinning.
3. **Note Patterns:** Which areas of the scalp thinned first? Was it the crown, temples, or a general spread?

Combining this research with a doctor's advice or a genetic test can give you a good sense of your starting point.

6.12 Epigenetics: More Than Just DNA

Epigenetics is the study of how behaviors or environmental factors can switch certain genes on or off. Even if someone has genes for hair loss, certain habits might speed it up or slow it down. For example, smoking, poor diet, or persistent stress could switch on certain pathways that negatively affect hair follicles, while healthy living might keep them calmer.

This does not mean you can completely stop the genetic process if you are highly prone to baldness. However, some men do see a slower or less noticeable thinning process when they adopt a balanced lifestyle and address any underlying health issues.

6.13 Genetic Factors in Other Hair Loss Types

Besides male pattern baldness, genetics can play a part in:

- **Alopecia Areata:** Some families have a higher incidence of this autoimmune condition.
- **Scarring Alopecia:** Certain inherited inflammatory conditions can lead to scarring of follicles.
- **Telogen Effluvium Tendency:** While stress is the main driver, a tendency to overreact to physical or emotional strain might run in families as well.

When you notice anything unusual, it is best to rule out these other causes by consulting a specialist. Genetic predisposition might raise the likelihood, but each condition often has unique triggers.

6.14 Myths About Family History and Hair Loss

- **Myth:** If your maternal grandfather was bald, you must be bald too.
  - **Fact:** While there may be a gene on the X chromosome, there are many other genes that might or might not be present.
- **Myth:** You can tell everything by your father's hair.
  - **Fact:** Both sides contribute genetic material, plus your environment matters.
- **Myth:** If you have no bald relatives, you will never lose hair.
  - **Fact:** It is possible to have a "new" mutation or a less obvious family history and still experience male pattern thinning.

6.15 When Family History Is Unclear

Sometimes, a man might not know much about his relatives' health. This could be due to adoption or because older generations did not discuss such issues. If you are in this position, you can still pay attention to your own hairline and any changes that pop up. If you have concerns, consider:

1. **Speaking with a Dermatologist:** They can do a thorough check and suggest tests.
2. **Keeping a Photo Journal:** Take pictures of your hair at regular intervals to spot any trends.
3. **Genetic Test Kits:** Though not perfect, they can shed some light on potential risk factors.

6.16 Combining Genes with Other Factors

Even with a strong genetic component, the actual experience of hair loss is often a mix of multiple elements:

- **Hormones:** High DHT or unusual thyroid activity may accelerate or exacerbate genetic tendencies.
- **Age:** The older you get, the greater the chance that any inherited trait may appear.
- **Health and Habits:** Poor diets or chronic stress can make hair loss worse, even if genes are mild.
- **Medical Conditions:** Issues such as autoimmune disorders might overlap with genetic traits, creating more severe hair loss.

6.17 Practical Steps if You Suspect Genetic Hair Loss

1. **Early Assessment:** If you see a receding hairline or thinning areas, consult a professional sooner rather than later.
2. **Lifestyle Upgrades:** Improve diet, manage stress, and exercise regularly to keep your body in better shape.
3. **Medications:** You can consider options like finasteride or minoxidil to slow or reduce genetic thinning, under a doctor's guidance.
4. **Surgical Options:** If hair loss is more advanced and bothersome, you might explore a hair transplant procedure in the future.
5. **Track Progress:** Keep an eye on whether treatments are working. Some men take regular photos to compare.

6.18 Real-World Examples

- **Family A:** The father has a full head of hair at 60, the mother's father lost most of his hair by 40. The son notices a slight thinning at 35. After a genetic test, he finds that he carries some markers for hair loss but at a moderate level. With minoxidil and healthy habits, he maintains decent coverage well into his 50s.
- **Family B:** No clear record of baldness on either side. Yet the son starts to see a receding hairline at 22. It turns out a great-grandparent on the paternal line had early baldness, and the trait skipped a few generations before showing up again.

6.19 The Future of Genetics in Hair Loss

As genetic research moves forward, we might see:

1. **Personalized Treatments:** Doctors selecting the best medication based on a person's genetic makeup.
2. **Preventive Approaches:** Identifying those at high risk and recommending early interventions.
3. **Gene Editing (in the Far Future):** Possibly adjusting hair-related genes to avoid scalp follicle shrinking.

We are not at that stage yet, but the field is advancing quickly. Understanding that genes are a crucial piece, but not the entire puzzle, can help men handle their hair loss concerns in a more informed way.

Chapter 7: Lifestyle Choices and Their Influence

Hair loss in men can sometimes be made worse or brought on sooner by daily habits. While genetics and hormones are strong reasons, the ways men live—what they eat, how they handle stress, and the types of products they use—can push hair toward a healthier state or one of greater risk. In many cases, changing certain patterns might not fully prevent hair loss, especially for those with a powerful genetic background. However, these changes can still make a notable difference in hair quality, scalp health, and the speed at which thinning occurs.

This chapter will focus on many lifestyle elements that can support or harm hair health. We will look at stress management, eating patterns, hydration, exercise, grooming methods, and more. By the end, you will see that the choices made each day can change how hair grows and whether it remains strong or becomes weak over time.

7.1 Stress and Hair Loss

7.1.1 Stress Hormones and the Hair Cycle

When a person is under stress, the body produces more cortisol. This is often known as the "stress hormone." High levels of cortisol for a long time can disturb many systems in the body, including the hair growth cycle. It may cause more hairs to enter the resting or shedding phase too soon, which is seen in conditions like telogen effluvium. While androgenetic alopecia is linked mainly to DHT, stress can still make thinning worse if combined with other factors.

7.1.2 Everyday Stress vs. High-Impact Events

Not all stress is the same. Mild, everyday stress—like meeting work deadlines—may not produce major changes in hair. More severe stress, such as losing a loved one, facing a major illness, or prolonged anxiety, can have a bigger impact. Men might see a noticeable increase in shedding a few weeks or months after these events.

7.1.3 Methods to Manage Stress

- **Relaxation Techniques:** Simple breathing exercises, stretching, or short breaks can help calm the mind.
- **Support Systems:** Talking to friends, family, or a counselor can ease emotional burdens.
- **Physical Activity:** Moderate exercise releases endorphins, which help counteract stress hormones.
- **Adequate Rest:** Sleep gives the body and scalp time to recover.

Although these tactics will not directly eliminate genetic hair loss, they can reduce one potential source of extra shedding.

7.2 The Role of Nutrition

7.2.1 Protein

Hair is mostly made of keratin, a protein-based structure. Eating enough protein helps the body maintain the building blocks required for healthy hair growth. Lean meats, fish, eggs, beans, and nuts are examples of good protein sources. If the body does not get enough protein, hair strands can weaken or look dull.

7.2.2 Vitamins and Minerals

Several vitamins and minerals are needed for healthy hair:

- **Vitamin A:** Helps produce natural oils that keep the scalp moisturized. However, too much Vitamin A can trigger shedding.
- **Vitamin C:** Needed for collagen production, which helps hair stay strong. Also aids iron absorption.
- **B Vitamins (including Biotin):** Support cell growth and can assist in preventing brittle strands.

- **Vitamin D:** Some studies link low Vitamin D to hair thinning. Sunlight is a natural source, but supplements and certain foods also help.
- **Iron:** Delivers oxygen to hair follicles. Low iron levels can lead to weak or thinning hair, especially in those with borderline anemia.
- **Zinc:** Important for repair processes in the scalp and for oil gland function around follicles.

7.2.3 Fatty Acids

Omega-3 fatty acids, found in foods like salmon, flaxseeds, and walnuts, can help reduce dryness and inflammation of the scalp. A balanced intake of healthy fats can contribute to a healthier hair appearance over time.

7.2.4 Moderation and Balance

Drastic diets or cutting out entire food groups without medical guidance may create nutrient gaps that affect hair. Rapid weight loss can cause temporary shedding because the body sees it as a form of stress. A balanced approach to eating, with consistent portions of protein, vegetables, fruits, whole grains, and healthy fats, can give hair a stable environment to grow.

7.3 Hydration for Hair Health

7.3.1 Why Water Matters

Hair follicles need adequate moisture, just like skin and other tissues. When a person is dehydrated, the body may channel water to vital organs first, possibly leaving the scalp under-hydrated. A dry scalp can become itchy, irritated, and prone to flaking.

7.3.2 Drinking Habits

There is no single rule on how much water a person needs, since factors like climate, physical activity level, and body size vary. However, a general recommendation is about 6 to 8 cups of fluid a day for an adult. Water-rich fruits and vegetables (like cucumbers or watermelon) can contribute to total hydration as well.

7.3.3 Moisture in the Scalp

Proper hydration helps produce natural oils that keep the scalp environment balanced. Over-shampooing or using harsh products may strip these oils, making hair more fragile. Maintaining a hydrated scalp through a proper water intake and mild hair care products can reduce breakage and may help hair keep a healthy shine.

7.4 Exercise and Hair Loss

7.4.1 Blood Circulation and Nutrient Delivery

Exercise helps pump blood throughout the body, including the scalp. Better circulation means nutrients can reach hair follicles more effectively. Activities like brisk walking, swimming, or light strength training can offer these benefits without raising stress hormones too much.

7.4.2 Overtraining and Stress

While moderate exercise is helpful, extreme workouts can push the body into high stress, increasing cortisol production. Some people also follow very restrictive diets to stay lean, which can deprive hair of necessary nutrients. This can become a source of hair weakening.

7.4.3 Practical Tips

- **Balance:** Aim for moderate workouts several times a week.
- **Variety:** Alternate between cardio and light strength exercises to avoid overuse injuries and burnout.
- **Rest Days:** The body, including the scalp, recovers when given time off from intense activity.

7.5 Harmful Habits: Smoking and Alcohol

7.5.1 Smoking

Cigarette smoke contains toxins that can reduce blood flow to hair follicles and damage hair at a cellular level. Smoking may also speed up the normal aging process, making hair look dull or prone to breakage. Studies show that smokers may see more rapid hair thinning compared to non-smokers with the same genetic risk.

7.5.2 Alcohol

Excessive alcohol intake can lead to nutrient shortages because the body focuses on removing alcohol and might not absorb vitamins and minerals effectively. Dehydration is another concern, as alcohol pulls water out of tissues. Over time, hair follicles can suffer from insufficient nutrition or dryness.

7.5.3 Reducing or Quitting

Cutting back on smoking or drinking, or giving them up entirely, can have positive effects on overall health and, by extension, hair. While it may not prevent male pattern baldness for those genetically prone, it can slow additional weakening or dryness that worsens thinning.

7.6 Hair Care Methods

7.6.1 Shampoo Choices

Many shampoos contain sulfates or other harsh cleansers that can irritate the scalp if used too often. Men with thinning hair may benefit from milder shampoos made for sensitive scalps. These products can help wash away excess oil and dirt without stripping the scalp's natural protective layer.

7.6.2 Conditioner and Scalp Treatments

Conditioners can add a protective film around each strand, helping to reduce breakage. Some men skip conditioner, thinking it is unnecessary, but using a lightweight version can make hair smoother and look fuller. Certain scalp treatments also aim to balance oils or reduce inflammation, although results can vary.

7.6.3 Styling Choices

Tight hair styles or constant pulling can cause traction alopecia. While men often do not wear tight braids or similar styles as frequently, hats or sports helmets might also exert tension. Moderation in wearing tight headgear can help reduce this risk.

7.6.4 Heat Tools

Using very hot tools, like strong blow dryers or hair straighteners, can damage hair shafts and lead to dryness or split ends. If possible, letting hair air-dry or using lower heat settings can keep hair healthier.

7.6.5 Chemicals and Dyes

Men who dye or bleach their hair frequently should note that these chemicals can weaken hair structure. Frequent or improper use can increase breakage and highlight thinning. If coloring hair is important, spacing out sessions and using quality products can minimize damage.

7.7 Environmental Factors

7.7.1 Pollution

Air pollutants, dust, and chemical particles in urban environments can settle on the scalp, combining with natural oils to form build-up. This might clog follicles if not cleaned properly. Gentle but regular washing can help remove these substances.

7.7.2 Sun Exposure

Overexposure to UV rays can harm the scalp. For men who already have thinning hair, the skin might be more exposed to sunlight, risking sunburn or dryness. Using hats (not overly tight) or a scalp-friendly sunscreen can reduce damage.

7.7.3 Workplace Hazards

Some jobs involve exposure to chemicals, oils, or extreme heat. Wearing protective gear or washing hair and scalp promptly after work helps reduce potential harm. Over time, repeated exposure to harsh substances can irritate or dry out the scalp.

7.8 Rest and Sleep

7.8.1 Importance of Sleep

During sleep, the body repairs tissues and balances hormones. Men with consistent, high-quality sleep often show healthier hair and skin. Without enough rest, hormones like cortisol may remain high, and cell repair may be limited, weakening hair shafts over time.

7.8.2 Sleep Disorders

Problems such as sleep apnea or chronic insomnia can increase stress on the body. If these are not addressed, they can contribute to hair shedding and slow regrowth. Men suspecting they have a sleep disorder may consider a medical checkup.

7.8.3 Tips for Better Rest

- **Set a Routine:** Going to bed at a similar time nightly can help regulate the internal clock.
- **Calm Environment:** Keep screens and bright lights away an hour before sleep if possible.

- **Moderate Caffeine:** Avoid coffee or tea late in the day, as they can disturb rest.

7.9 Grooming Habits That Can Weaken Hair

1. **Over-Brushing:** Excessive or rough brushing can cause breakage, especially if hair is already thin. Using a wide-toothed comb or a soft-bristle brush gently can help.
2. **Frequent Shampooing:** Washing once a day or every other day can be enough for most men, depending on scalp oiliness. Washing too frequently with harsh products might strip natural oils.
3. **Hot Showers:** Very hot water can dry the scalp. Warm or lukewarm water is often gentler.
4. **Rubbing Hair Dry:** Vigorous towel-drying can pull on strands. Patting hair dry is easier on the scalp.

7.10 Avoiding Sudden Lifestyle Changes

Some men try crash diets or suddenly switch to very intense workouts. Such dramatic changes can be a shock to the body. Rapid weight loss sometimes triggers telogen effluvium. Big shifts in exercise might spike cortisol. It is often better to make slow, gradual changes that the body can handle without going into a stress response.

7.11 Golden Tidbits and Lesser-Known Facts

- **Scalp Tension Theory:** Some experts suggest that tension in scalp muscles might limit blood flow to hair follicles, making hair more prone to shedding in certain patterns. Stretching or light scalp massage might loosen these muscles and help with circulation.
- **Saltwater and Chlorine:** Regular swimming in the ocean or pools can dry out hair and scalp, so rinsing thoroughly afterward is wise.

- **Heated Environments:** Jobs in very warm settings (like kitchens) might raise scalp oil production, leading to frequent washing that could irritate hair unless a gentle product is used.

7.12 Combining Lifestyle Strategies with Medical Care

Lifestyle adjustments alone may not stop hair loss for men with a strong genetic or hormonal component. However, adopting healthy habits can strengthen hair that is still growing and may slow the rate of thinning. In many cases, doctors who prescribe treatments such as minoxidil or finasteride also advise patients to work on stress reduction, balanced eating, and proper scalp care.

Treating hair loss often involves a combined plan:

1. **Medical or pharmaceutical methods** (if needed).
2. **Lifestyle changes** that give hair a better foundation.
3. **Regular scalp monitoring** to see if the problem is stabilizing.

7.13 Creating a Personal Routine

Each person is unique. What works best for one may not work as well for another. Some men might find they need to shampoo daily due to an oily scalp, while others do fine with every-other-day washing. Similarly, one man's stress might come from an intense work environment, while another may feel more pressure from personal issues. Recognizing personal triggers and adjusting accordingly can help hair stay in better shape.

A simple plan might include:

- Drinking enough water throughout the day.
- Having a balanced breakfast that includes protein.
- Doing moderate exercise 3-4 times a week.
- Practicing a 5-minute relaxation exercise before bedtime.

- Using a mild shampoo and conditioner.

Over time, keeping track of changes in hair thickness or scalp comfort helps show if these efforts are making a difference.

7.14 Psychological Benefits of a Positive Lifestyle

Taking better care of one's body and hair can also have emotional benefits. Many men feel more confident when they know they are making constructive lifestyle decisions. This can lower stress, which further supports hair health. In this sense, healthy habits become a feedback loop that supports both physical and mental well-being.

7.15 Technology and Lifestyle Tracking

Some men use smartphone apps or wearable devices to monitor sleep, steps taken, or heart rate. While these do not directly track hair growth, they can reveal patterns in stress or physical activity. If you notice that your hair loss spikes after periods of poor sleep or extreme workouts, the data might encourage you to adjust your schedule.

Chapter 8: The TrichoTest (Genetic Testing for Hair Loss)

In the area of men's hair loss, genetic screening has grown in importance. The TrichoTest is a cutting-edge test designed to provide clear insights into the genetic reasons behind hair thinning. By analyzing specific markers in a person's genetic code, it aims to predict how hair follicles may react to hormones, medications, and treatment approaches.

This chapter explains what the TrichoTest is, how it works, and who might benefit from it. We will also look at the potential benefits and any drawbacks. While it is not a magic tool that cures hair loss, the TrichoTest is a new option in personalizing care for men dealing with thinning or receding hair.

8.1 Basics of Genetic Hair Testing

In recent years, genetic testing has become more accessible. A person provides a sample of their DNA—usually through saliva or a cheek swab—and a lab examines certain markers. For hair loss, these markers relate to genes involved in hair growth cycles, sensitivity to DHT, and other aspects.

8.1.1 What Sets the TrichoTest Apart?

The TrichoTest focuses on multiple gene variants known to influence hair loss. It tries to capture a wide range of factors, from how a body handles inflammation to how quickly it breaks down hormones. Unlike a broad ancestry test that checks large segments of DNA for heritage details, the TrichoTest zeroes in on hair health.

8.2 Who Should Consider the TrichoTest?

1. **Men in Early Stages of Hair Thinning:** If someone sees the first signs of a receding hairline in their twenties or thirties, the TrichoTest could show how likely it is to advance.
2. **Those with Family History:** Men whose relatives had severe or early pattern baldness might want to see if they share the same genetic markers.
3. **Not Responding to Standard Treatments:** If a person has used finasteride or minoxidil for months with little benefit, the test might reveal if their genetic setup is resistant to these treatments.
4. **Anyone Planning a Long-Term Hair Care Strategy:** The test can help doctors create a more personalized approach.

8.3 How the Test is Done

8.3.1 Sample Collection

A basic kit is provided. The user typically swabs the inside of their cheek or spits into a small tube. The kit is then sealed and mailed to the testing lab.

8.3.2 Laboratory Analysis

The lab extracts DNA from the sample. It then examines specific genetic markers connected to hair growth, hormone sensitivity, and scalp health. This is often done using technologies like PCR (Polymerase Chain Reaction) or microarray chips designed for hair-related genes.

8.3.3 Results Report

After a few weeks, the lab sends a report showing which markers are present. The report often includes a risk scale or a summary of how those markers might affect hair loss. Some labs also suggest which treatments may fit best with the person's genetic profile, such as indicating whether finasteride is likely to be more or less helpful.

8.4 Interpreting the Results

While the TrichoTest can point to certain genetic tendencies, it cannot guarantee a specific outcome. Having a high-risk gene might raise the chances of early or severe hair loss, but it does not mean it will certainly happen at a given time. Likewise, testing low risk does not mean hair will never thin.

Clinics usually recommend discussing the report with a dermatologist or a hair specialist. These professionals can explain how each genetic marker may play out given the individual's lifestyle, hormone levels, and health history. This helps avoid misreading the data and jumping to wrong conclusions.

8.5 Possible Benefits of the TrichoTest

1. **Personalized Treatment:** If the report shows a strong sensitivity to DHT, the person might focus on finasteride or other DHT-blocking methods. If the test indicates a lower response to minoxidil, the individual might try a different topical approach or combine minoxidil with other therapies.
2. **Early Intervention:** Men who know they are at high risk can start preventive steps sooner, possibly slowing the process of hair loss.
3. **Targeted Lifestyle Changes:** Some markers might hint at a bigger role of inflammation or nutritional factors, guiding men to pay extra attention to diet or scalp care.
4. **Confidence in Decisions:** Instead of guessing, a man might feel more assured choosing treatments backed by his genetic profile.

8.6 Potential Drawbacks and Limitations

1. **Cost:** The TrichoTest can be more expensive than standard medical consultations. Not all insurance plans cover it.

2. **Availability:** It may not be available in all areas, and shipping samples to certain countries can be complex.
3. **False Sense of Certainty:** Genetics is only part of the puzzle. Stress, diet, and other conditions also matter. A person could place too much trust in the test results and ignore other factors.
4. **Privacy:** Storing genetic data can raise questions about how labs use or protect this information. Individuals should read the privacy policies carefully.

8.7 Comparing TrichoTest to General Genetic Tests

Not all genetic tests are the same. Some direct-to-consumer kits give broad overviews of health traits or ancestry, with a small focus on hair loss. The TrichoTest, on the other hand, is specialized. It may look at a larger number of hair-related markers, offering more detailed insight about how an individual's scalp might respond to common treatments.

That said, the accuracy and usefulness of any genetic test depends on how thoroughly those genes were studied and validated. Quality labs will publish data on the scientific basis for each gene they include. Checking these references or asking a medical professional about them can help a user gauge how reliable the test is.

8.8 Using TrichoTest Results for Treatment

8.8.1 Finasteride or Dutasteride

If the TrichoTest shows that a person's follicles are highly sensitive to DHT, a doctor might discuss finasteride or dutasteride. These drugs block the enzyme that converts testosterone to DHT. The test might hint if the user has a higher risk of side effects or if the drug is likely to be effective.

8.8.2 Minoxidil

Some men have gene markers that suggest a reduced response to minoxidil. They might decide to use a higher-strength version, combine it with other treatments, or look at alternatives like low-level laser therapy.

8.8.3 Anti-Inflammatory Approaches

If the test suggests a role for inflammation in that person's hair loss, the plan may involve medicated shampoos, topical steroids, or diet adjustments to reduce inflammatory triggers.

8.8.4 Nutritional Guidance

Certain genetic markers can reveal whether the body has trouble absorbing or using specific nutrients. In these cases, a physician or nutritionist might advise specialized supplements or changes in meal planning to support hair growth.

8.9 Personal Stories and Outcomes

1. **Case A:** A 28-year-old with mild recession learns through the TrichoTest that he has high DHT sensitivity but a favorable response marker for finasteride. He starts the medication early, sees limited side effects, and stabilizes his hairline for several years.
2. **Case B:** Another man has tried minoxidil without success. The TrichoTest shows he lacks certain markers for strong minoxidil response. He switches to a laser therapy routine plus finasteride and notices better results after six months.
3. **Case C:** A user with moderate thinning discovers that he is prone to scalp inflammation. He adds special anti-inflammatory shampoos to his routine along with standard medication, which improves his scalp condition and reduces irritation-related shedding.

These examples illustrate how the test can direct men toward solutions that fit their genetic profiles.

8.10 Ethical and Privacy Questions

Collecting genetic data comes with responsibilities. Users should confirm what happens to their DNA sample after the test is done:

- Will it be stored for future research?
- Are the results shared with third parties?
- Can the user request deletion of their genetic profile from the lab's systems?

Transparency is crucial. Reputable labs outline their privacy policies and allow customers to ask questions about data handling. When in doubt, men should talk to a doctor or pharmacist who is knowledgeable about the test and any local laws on genetic privacy.

8.11 How TrichoTest Fits Into a Wider Hair Loss Plan

The TrichoTest is not a stand-alone fix. It should be viewed as one piece of information among many. Doctors still look at hormones, scalp condition, patient age, stress levels, and family history when forming a treatment plan. Lifestyle adjustments (as explained in Chapter 7) remain important.

The true advantage of the TrichoTest is in shaping a more individualized approach. Men who have tried a one-size-fits-all path might find that aligning treatments with their genetic markers yields better outcomes. Yet it is also important to keep realistic expectations. Even with precise data, hair loss might continue if the genetic drive is strong.

8.12 Potential Future Developments

Research on hair-related genes is ongoing. As scientists identify new markers, the TrichoTest or similar tests may expand to cover more variants.

We could see deeper analysis of scalp microbes or epigenetic factors that influence how genes work. Another angle might be discovering markers that predict who will respond best to emerging therapies like stem cell transplants or hair cloning (which are still experimental).

For now, men who are curious about their genetic makeup can consider the TrichoTest, keeping in mind that it is one tool in a growing toolkit of modern hair loss evaluations.

8.13 Cost Considerations

Prices for the TrichoTest can range widely depending on location and specific lab. Some clinics bundle the test with a consultation and interpretation of results. Others require the user to pay separately for the kit and for any follow-up medical advice. Insurance coverage varies; many health plans do not cover genetic hair loss tests because they see it as a quality-of-life or cosmetic matter.

Men should compare prices, read reviews, and discuss options with healthcare providers. A cheaper test might still offer valuable insights, but it is good to ensure that the lab is reputable and has a reliable track record in analyzing hair loss genetics.

8.14 Combining TrichoTest with Other Assessments

Beyond genetics, a comprehensive hair loss workup might include:

1. **Blood Tests:** Checking iron levels, thyroid hormones, and other possible deficiencies.
2. **Hormone Profile:** Measuring testosterone, DHT, and others if needed.
3. **Scalp Exam:** A physical check can spot inflammation, scaling, or other signs of non-genetic hair loss conditions.

4. **Family History Discussion:** Seeing if the pattern matches close relatives.

Putting all these pieces together provides the best view of what is happening and how to address it.

8.15 Common Questions About the TrichoTest

1. Will the test tell me exactly when I will go bald?
No. It only gives a sense of genetic likelihood. Other factors also affect the speed and pattern of hair loss.

2. Do I have to see a doctor to get the test?
Some clinics require a prescription or an official request from a medical professional. Others allow direct purchases. However, getting a doctor's help to interpret the results is often recommended.

3. Is the test painful?
Not at all. The usual sample collection involves swabbing the inside of the cheek or spitting into a tube.

4. Do I need the TrichoTest if I already know my family history shows baldness?
It can still help by showing how you might respond to certain treatments or if you have additional markers for inflammation. But if you prefer not to have genetic testing, you can still try common treatments under a doctor's supervision.

8.16 Tips for Making the Most of the TrichoTest

1. **Choose a Trusted Provider:** Make sure the lab performing the test is known for quality results and good data handling practices.
2. **Plan a Consultation:** Have a specialist explain the data. This reduces confusion about what the numbers or markers mean.

3. **Keep Expectations Realistic:** Even if you learn you are a strong responder to minoxidil, you might not see a total reversal of hair loss.
4. **Pair with a Balanced Lifestyle:** Continue focusing on nutrition, stress management, and scalp care. Genetics is not everything.
5. **Monitor Results Over Time:** Keep track of your hair's thickness or hairline changes every few months. Genetic info is a starting point, but the real test is how your scalp responds in daily life.

8.17 Could the Test Prevent a Hair Transplant?

For some men, the TrichoTest results may encourage them to try or stick with treatments longer before considering a hair transplant. If the test shows high potential for good response to medication, a transplant might be postponed or avoided. However, for men with advanced hair loss, a transplant could still be on the table. The genetic test might help plan the best medication regimen to protect both existing hair and transplanted grafts over the long run.

Chapter 9: Non-Medical Tips for Managing Hair Loss

Men often look for ways to handle hair loss without turning to medication right away. Some prefer to try home methods or gentle approaches before deciding on more advanced treatments. Others use non-medical options together with medical approaches to get better outcomes. Either way, there are many strategies that can help give the hair a fuller look or slow down the process of thinning.

In this chapter, we will look at non-medical tips for dealing with hair loss. We will cover general grooming ideas, specific hair care tools, simple home routines, everyday habits, mental well-being tips, and more. While these suggestions may not stop true genetic hair loss, they can improve how hair looks and possibly make thinning less obvious.

9.1 Understanding the Limits of Non-Medical Methods

It is helpful to know that non-medical methods do not always tackle the root causes of hair loss, especially if hormones or genetics are behind it. However, these methods can still help hair appear thicker or keep the scalp in better shape. For many men, these approaches can be an early step before trying medicine or surgery.

Some men also find it useful to combine non-medical tips with other solutions. For example, a person might follow a certain styling technique along with using a topical solution. Doing so can give a balanced approach, addressing both appearance and underlying factors.

9.2 Good Grooming Basics

9.2.1 Gentle Washing Techniques

Using a mild shampoo helps remove excess oil and dirt without stripping the scalp of important protective oils. Over-washing can lead to dryness and cause hair to break more easily. On the other hand, not washing enough might lead to buildup that can weigh hair down and make thinning more noticeable.

- **Choose a Mild Shampoo:** Look for products labeled for frequent or daily use.
- **Lukewarm Water:** Hot water can irritate the scalp and weaken hair strands.
- **Soft Toweling:** Pat hair dry instead of rubbing it to avoid tugging on weakened follicles.

9.2.2 Conditioner

Conditioner can add a slight protective layer around each strand, reducing friction when combing or brushing. This can be beneficial for thin or fragile hair. Some conditioners also include proteins or vitamins that can give hair a smoother look.

- **Apply to Ends Primarily:** Focus on the tips of the hair, where dryness is most common.
- **Avoid the Roots if Oily:** Men with oily scalps may want to avoid applying conditioner directly on the roots.

9.2.3 Comb vs. Brush

Wide-toothed combs or soft brushes can reduce pulling on the scalp. Avoid yanking out knots too aggressively. Starting at the ends and slowly working upward can untangle hair with less damage.

9.3 Styling Tips to Create a Fuller Look

9.3.1 Haircuts Suited for Thinning Hair

Choosing the right hairstyle can make a big difference. Shorter haircuts often make thinning less obvious because there is not a strong contrast between the hair and the scalp. In some cases, a fade on the sides can draw attention away from the top.

Many barbers are experienced with styling thinning hair. Explaining concerns to a barber can allow them to suggest specific cuts that add the illusion of volume or reduce visible scalp in problem areas.

9.3.2 Using Hair Fibers

Hair fiber products are small, fine particles that cling to existing hair to create the effect of thicker coverage. They come in various colors to blend with natural hair shade. Once applied, they often stay in place until the next wash, though heavy sweat or rain can sometimes cause them to run or clump.

For some men, hair fibers are a convenient way to hide thinning spots, especially for social events or photos. They will not halt the underlying causes of hair loss, but they can improve appearance in a quick and easy way.

9.3.3 Volumizing Products

Special shampoos or mousses marketed as "volumizing" can help hair stand up a bit more, giving a fuller look. Be mindful not to use products containing harsh chemicals or heavy waxes, as these can build up over time and weigh the hair down.

9.4 Helpful Tools and Devices

9.4.1 Low-Level Light Devices (Home Use)

While formal clinic-based laser treatments fall partly under medical categories, there are also consumer-grade laser caps or combs available for home use. They use low-level light to stimulate blood flow to the scalp. Some men feel they benefit from these devices, though results are not uniform for everyone.

9.4.2 Scalp Massagers

Simple scalp massagers made of rubber or soft plastic can increase blood circulation to some extent. They can also help distribute natural oils across the scalp, which might support healthier strands. Regular, gentle use can also be soothing, helping reduce stress.

9.4.3 Silk or Satin Pillowcases

Rough pillowcase materials might increase friction on the hair and lead to tangles or breakage. Switching to silk or satin can lower friction, which may benefit those with delicate strands. While this does not fix hair loss, it can minimize hair shaft damage.

9.5 Home Routines and Practices

9.5.1 Warm Oil Treatments

Using natural oils like coconut oil or olive oil can bring moisture to the scalp. These oils contain fatty acids that can penetrate the hair shaft to some extent. A basic routine might involve warming the oil slightly (not too hot), massaging it into the scalp, leaving it on for 20-30 minutes, then rinsing it out thoroughly.

Some men add a few drops of essential oils, like rosemary or peppermint, which may help circulation or have mild antimicrobial effects. However, these are not proven cures. The main benefit is often softer, smoother hair that looks less frizzy.

9.5.2 Aloe-Based Gels or Masks

Aloe gel can be soothing for scalp irritation. Some people find it helpful for itching or mild redness. It will not make new hair grow in areas where follicles are shut down, but it can maintain a calmer scalp environment, which might help the existing hair look healthier.

9.5.3 Gentle Steam

A warm steam session (such as a warm shower with the bathroom door closed to trap steam) can open pores on the scalp briefly and make it easier for some conditioner or oil treatments to penetrate. This is a mild method that can be calming. Just be sure not to use water that is too hot, since that can do more harm than good.

9.6 Wearing Hats or Head Coverings

Some men worry that wearing hats too often causes hair to fall out faster. Generally, a normal-fitting hat does not harm follicles. What can be a problem is if the hat is extremely tight, leading to traction on the hair or limiting airflow, which might irritate the scalp.

- **Choose Breathable Materials:** Cotton or other breathable fabrics can reduce sweat and irritation.
- **Proper Fit:** A hat should not create strong pressure around the scalp.
- **Keep Hats Clean:** Dirty hats can lead to scalp irritation or infections.

If thinning is a concern for appearance, hats can serve as a simple way to hide the scalp on certain days. Some men feel more at ease in social situations when wearing a cap or beanie.

9.7 Stress and Emotional Support

Non-medical methods also include addressing how hair loss impacts mental well-being. Some men feel worried, sad, or frustrated about hair changes. Ignoring these feelings can add more stress, which may worsen the situation if stress-related shedding is part of the problem.

9.7.1 Talking to Friends or Family

Sometimes, sharing concerns about hair loss with trusted people can lift a burden. They might offer reassurance or practical suggestions. It can also help to realize that many men face the same problem and that it is not as noticeable to others as one might think.

9.7.2 Relaxation Methods

Simple breathing exercises, light meditation, or mild physical activities (like walking in a calm setting) can help reduce stress. When stress is lower, the body may function better overall, and the scalp environment could benefit as well.

9.7.3 Professional Counseling

If anxiety or self-esteem issues become overwhelming, speaking with a counselor or therapist could offer useful tools for coping. While it does not directly regrow hair, feeling more at peace can improve one's approach to hair care and life in general.

9.8 Nutrition Checks and Supplements (Non-Prescription)

A balanced diet is important for hair health. While we talked about general eating habits in a previous chapter, we can focus here on how men might use over-the-counter supplements.

- **Multivitamins:** Some men use these if they suspect their diet lacks certain nutrients.
- **Hair-Focused Supplements:** Many brands advertise formulas with ingredients like biotin, zinc, and collagen. These might help if someone is deficient, but they are not guaranteed to reverse genetic hair loss.
- **Protein Powders or Shakes:** If a person does not get enough protein from meals, adding a moderate amount of protein supplements can support the keratin structure of hair.

Still, it is wise to be cautious with high-dose supplements. Getting too much of certain nutrients (for instance, Vitamin A) can worsen shedding. Moderation and, if possible, guidance from a nutrition professional are recommended.

9.9 Avoiding Overly Harsh Chemicals

9.9.1 Hair Dyes and Bleaches

Frequent use of strong dyes or bleaches can break down the hair shaft, leading to splits and breakage. While this damage differs from genetic thinning, it can make hair look weaker. If coloring hair is desired, spacing out sessions or choosing gentler formulas can reduce harm.

9.9.2 Chemical Straighteners

Some men straighten hair to control curls or frizz. Strong chemical relaxers can be tough on hair, especially if left on too long or applied incorrectly. If hair is already thinning, the added stress might speed breakage. Choosing mild methods or professional salon services can reduce risks.

9.10 Protective Hairstyles and Routine Adjustments

While men's hairstyles vary widely, some do wear braids or tight buns. If these styles put strain on the scalp (traction), it can lead to traction alopecia over time. A looser style that does not pull at the roots is safer.

Similarly, adjusting daily routines can help:

- **Switch Sides:** If you part your hair on the same side for decades, that area might get worn. Changing the part occasionally can distribute tension more evenly.
- **Limit Heat Styling:** If you use a blow dryer or flat iron daily, try cutting back to a few times a week or using lower heat settings.

9.11 Scalp Hygiene and Possible Issues

Keeping the scalp clean is important, but it is also possible to overdo it. Striking the right balance may help keep follicles clear of buildup:

- **Mild Exfoliation:** Some products or homemade scrubs can gently remove dead skin cells. Overuse or harsh scrubs can lead to irritation, so moderation is key.
- **Identify Scalp Problems:** Conditions like dandruff, psoriasis, or fungal infections might worsen shedding if not treated. A special shampoo or mild medicated treatment could keep the scalp healthier.

9.12 Temporary Cosmetics and Covers

Aside from hair fibers, there are sprays and concealers that color the scalp slightly to match hair color. These can minimize the contrast between hair and scalp, making thinning areas less visible. Some come in powder form that clings to the hair, while others are liquid or spray-on. They often wash out with shampoo.

Such products are especially useful for events like weddings or important meetings. While they do not improve hair thickness biologically, they provide a quick fix for cosmetic appearance.

9.13 Posture and Appearance

Interestingly, posture and body language can affect how others perceive someone's hair. Standing upright with confidence can shift the focus away from the scalp. Slouching or tilting the head forward might highlight the top of the head, where thinning is more visible.

This does not stop hair loss, but it can change how you feel about your appearance and how others notice it. Confidence can also reduce stress, creating a small but helpful cycle of positivity.

9.14 Tracking Progress

Keeping track of changes can help men evaluate whether their non-medical methods are helping. Ways to track progress include:

- **Photos:** Taking pictures of the hairline or crown under similar lighting every few months.
- **Notes:** Writing down when scalp irritation flares or if shedding seems heavier.
- **Comparisons Over Time:** Looking back at older photos after six months or a year can reveal subtle improvements or further thinning.

This information can also be shared with a barber or dermatologist if medical help is sought later.

9.15 Social Support Groups

Some communities or online forums bring together people facing hair loss. Individuals share tips, product reviews, and emotional support. These groups can be a source of new ideas for non-medical methods or ways to style hair.

However, one must be careful with unproven "miracle cures" or spammy product links that sometimes appear in these groups. Always evaluate claims critically. If something sounds too good to be true, it likely is.

9.16 Professional Services Beyond Medicine

There are non-medical professionals who specialize in hair and scalp care, such as trichologists. They can offer analysis of hair structure, scalp condition, and daily habits. They might recommend certain changes or products that support healthier hair. Trichologists are not medical doctors, but they can be valuable if you want guidance that focuses on scalp health, styling, and gentle methods.

9.17 Using Wigs or Hairpieces

For men who have lost a lot of hair, wigs or hairpieces can be a non-medical way to achieve a desired appearance. Modern hair systems can look quite natural if they are of good quality and properly fitted.

- **Synthetic vs. Human Hair:** Synthetic pieces are usually cheaper and need less maintenance. Human hair pieces can look more natural but cost more.
- **Attachment Methods:** Some use adhesive tapes, clips, or bonding solutions. The durability varies, and removing them periodically to clean the scalp is important to avoid skin problems.

While some men are hesitant about wigs, others find them a helpful solution that does not require medicine or surgery. It is a personal choice based on comfort and preference.

9.18 Time and Consistency

Many non-medical methods require patience and regular effort. For instance, using a certain scalp massage or applying a product once a week will not show huge changes immediately. It might take weeks or months to see subtle benefits. If progress is not visible right away, that does not always mean the method is useless. Sometimes, small steps add up over time.

9.19 Realistic Expectations

Non-medical tips can make hair look better cared for, protect existing strands, and sometimes add slight thickness or reduce breakage. They do not usually regrow hair on bald spots that have been empty for years. Understanding this helps avoid feeling frustrated or misled.

That said, a good routine can extend the life of your current hair and keep the scalp in good condition, especially if you are also considering or already using medical interventions.

Chapter 10: Medical Treatments and Medications

While many men choose to start with non-medical tips, there are times when medical treatments become a stronger option to manage hair loss. Advances in research have given rise to several medications and clinical procedures that address hair thinning at deeper levels. Some treatments aim to block hormones that cause hair shrinkage, while others try to enhance hair follicle activity.

In this chapter, we will discuss the major medical treatments used to fight male hair loss, what they do, possible side effects, and points to think about when deciding whether to use them. We will also examine how doctors often pair treatments for better outcomes and what to watch out for when seeking professional guidance.

10.1 Why Consider Medical Treatments?

Genetic hair loss, also called androgenetic alopecia, has a strong link to hormones like DHT. Non-medical methods can help with appearance, but they usually do not stop this hormonal process. That is where medical approaches come in. They can slow or block the action of DHT, extend the active growth phase of hair, or otherwise protect the follicles.

Men who seek medical solutions often do so because:

- They want a longer-term strategy to slow or stabilize genetic thinning.
- They have tried non-medical steps and want extra help.
- They feel distressed by rapid or visible hair loss and want a more targeted solution.

10.2 Finasteride (Oral Medication)

10.2.1 How It Works

Finasteride is one of the most commonly known medications for male pattern baldness. It reduces the enzyme 5-alpha reductase, which is responsible for converting testosterone to DHT. By lowering DHT levels in the scalp, finasteride can help stop the shrinking of follicles in men who are prone to this process.

10.2.2 Benefits

- Slowing or even halting hair loss in many men.
- Some experience modest regrowth, mainly at the crown.
- Generally easy to take (a once-daily pill).

10.2.3 Potential Side Effects

- Changes in sex drive or function (reduced desire or mild performance issues), though not all users have this.
- Rare mood changes.
- Some men notice no side effects at all.

It usually takes three to six months to see visible changes. If stopped, hair loss often resumes. Checking with a doctor about side effects and keeping track of any changes is important.

10.3 Dutasteride

Dutasteride, similar to finasteride, also blocks 5-alpha reductase. In fact, it blocks both types of the enzyme (Type I and II), whereas finasteride primarily blocks Type II. Some researchers believe dutasteride can be more potent in reducing DHT.

- **Usage:** Often considered when finasteride is not showing enough results or if a doctor suspects both enzyme types are highly active.

- **Side Effects:** Can be similar to those of finasteride (changes in sex drive, mood, etc.).
- **Availability:** In some regions, it might not be approved or is used "off-label" for hair loss.

10.4 Minoxidil (Topical Treatment)

10.4.1 Mechanism of Action

Minoxidil was first a blood pressure medication. It was later noticed that it could encourage hair growth. When applied to the scalp, it can dilate blood vessels, possibly improving follicle nutrition and prolonging the growth phase of hair.

10.4.2 Application and Forms

Minoxidil usually comes in a liquid or foam. Men apply it once or twice a day directly to thinning areas. Massaging it gently helps spread it around the scalp.

- **Concentration:** There are 2% and 5% versions. The 5% is more common for men.
- **Alcohol Content:** Some formulas have alcohol, which can dry the scalp, while others have less alcohol for sensitive skin.

10.4.3 Expected Results

- **Slowing Hair Loss:** Many men see reduced shedding within a few months.
- **Possible Regrowth:** Some men notice small new hairs, especially at the crown.
- **Commitment:** Stopping minoxidil usually leads to loss of the gained or preserved hair.

10.4.4 Side Effects

- Mild itching or dryness of the scalp.

- Rarely, increased facial hair if the solution runs down the forehead or is absorbed beyond the scalp area.

10.5 Combining Finasteride and Minoxidil

Doctors sometimes prescribe both finasteride (to block DHT) and minoxidil (to help follicles grow more actively). These two medications work in different ways, so using them together can give broader coverage. Some men find better results with this combination than with either treatment alone.

- **Routine:** Oral finasteride once daily + minoxidil applied topically once or twice a day.
- **Monitoring:** Doctors advise checking progress every few months to decide if dosage changes or additional treatments are needed.

10.6 Topical Finasteride

Some newer products blend finasteride into a topical solution, aiming to deliver the drug directly to the scalp. Advocates suggest that this could reduce the chance of systemic side effects, like changes in sex drive, since less finasteride enters the bloodstream. However, studies are ongoing, and the safety profile is still being established.

- **Usage:** Applied similarly to minoxidil.
- **Availability:** Might be limited, and some formulas are made by specialized compounding pharmacies.
- **Effectiveness:** Early reports are promising, but it is not yet as widely used or researched as oral finasteride.

10.7 Low-Level Laser Therapy (Clinical Sessions)

Beyond home-use devices, there are clinical laser systems that deliver consistent low-level light therapy. These sessions are usually administered once or twice a week, and each session can last about 15 to 30 minutes.

- **Goal:** Increase blood flow to follicles, reduce inflammation, and boost cellular activity.
- **Limits:** Not all men respond well. It can be costly and time-consuming.
- **Combination:** Often used alongside medications for improved results.

10.8 Platelet-Rich Plasma (PRP)

PRP involves taking a small amount of the patient's blood, spinning it in a centrifuge to concentrate platelets, and then injecting that into thinning areas of the scalp. The growth factors in platelets might help follicles work better.

- **Sessions:** Typically repeated every month or two, for a series of treatments.
- **Results:** Some men notice thicker or stronger hair, but outcomes vary widely.
- **Drawbacks:** Can be expensive, and may cause some scalp tenderness after injections.

10.9 Steroid Injections for Autoimmune Conditions

If hair loss is due to conditions like alopecia areata (an immune system attack on follicles), doctors sometimes use steroid injections in small areas of hair loss. This reduces local inflammation, allowing hair to grow again.

- **Use Case:** Patchy bald spots rather than classic male pattern thinning.
- **Frequency:** Injections every few weeks, adjusted based on response.
- **Risks:** Overuse can cause skin thinning or other local side effects.

10.10 Specialized Shampoos and Topical Treatments

Certain medicated shampoos contain ingredients like ketoconazole or other mild anti-androgens. Though not as strong as oral medications, they may help reduce scalp irritation, remove fungal issues, or slightly lower DHT at the surface level.

- **Ketoconazole Shampoo:** Sometimes used twice a week. It can reduce scalp problems and might offer a mild effect on DHT.
- **Steroid Scalp Lotions:** Prescribed if there is redness or dermatitis that could worsen shedding.

These are typically not strong enough alone to tackle genetic hair loss but can complement more potent treatments.

10.11 Hair Transplants

A hair transplant is a surgical method where follicles from the back or sides of the scalp (where hair is usually resistant to DHT) are moved to thinning or bald areas. Two main techniques are used:

1. **FUT (Follicular Unit Transplantation):** A strip of scalp is removed from the donor area, then follicles are separated and transplanted.
2. **FUE (Follicular Unit Extraction):** Individual follicles are taken directly from the donor area using small punches, then inserted into the target spots.

10.11.1 Benefits

- Natural hair growth in the transplanted area.
- Long-lasting solution, because donor hairs are often resistant to DHT.
- Can significantly improve the look of a receding hairline or bald spot.

10.11.2 Drawbacks

- Surgery cost can be high.
- Recovery time and the possibility of scarring, depending on the technique.
- Does not stop future hair loss in non-transplanted areas, so ongoing medication might be needed.

10.11.3 Ideal Candidates

Men with stable hair loss patterns, good donor hair, and realistic goals often see the best results. Younger men with aggressive, ongoing hair loss might need a long-term plan that includes medicine before or after a transplant.

10.12 Scalp Micropigmentation

This method involves tattooing tiny dots on the scalp to resemble hair stubble or add the illusion of density between existing hairs. It does not regrow hair but can reduce the contrast between hair and skin, making thin areas look fuller or giving a "shaved head" look that appears thicker.

- **Procedure:** A professional uses specialized ink and tools. Usually done over multiple sessions to get the right shade and coverage.
- **Upkeep:** Fades over time, so touch-ups might be needed every few years.
- **Not Actual Hair:** Since it is a tattoo, it does not feel like hair to the touch, but it can look quite realistic from a short distance.

10.13 Emerging Therapies

10.13.1 Hair Cloning and Stem Cells

Researchers are studying ways to clone hair follicles or use stem cells to grow new follicles in a lab. If successful, these could provide an unlimited supply of donor hair for transplants or even direct follicle injections.

- **Status:** Mostly in experimental stages.
- **Future Potential:** Could be a major breakthrough, but real-world use might still be years away.

10.13.2 Gene-Based Treatments

Scientists are also exploring gene-editing tools that might switch off harmful signals in hair follicles. While this is promising, it remains very experimental with no current release date.

10.14 Risks and Considerations

Every medical option comes with potential downsides. Men should discuss these details with a certified dermatologist or hair specialist:

- **Side Effects:** Whether it is medication or surgery, weigh the pros and cons.
- **Duration and Cost:** Some treatments need ongoing payments and time investments.
- **Realistic Goals:** Medications might keep hair stable but not always create dramatic regrowth on large bald areas. Transplants can help, but require a healthy donor area.

10.15 Importance of Expert Guidance

A trained doctor can diagnose the exact type of hair loss and recommend the best medical approach. They might do blood tests, check scalp health, and examine family history before suggesting something like finasteride or a transplant.

Seeing an expert also helps avoid wasted money on treatments that do not match the diagnosis. For instance, a man with scarring alopecia might not benefit from standard DHT blockers if scarring is the main problem.

10.16 Follow-Up and Maintenance

Medical treatments for hair loss often require maintenance:

- **Finasteride or Minoxidil:** Must continue use to keep the benefits. Stopping can cause a return to previous patterns.
- **Laser Therapy or PRP:** Might need regular sessions to keep up any gains.
- **Transplants:** The transplanted hair is permanent, but surrounding native hair could still thin over time, so doctors often suggest continuing medication.

Regular follow-up visits can track results and tweak the plan if shedding speeds up or if new areas begin thinning.

10.17 Psychological Impact of Medical Treatments

Some men feel a boost in confidence once they see results from medication or surgery. But it is also possible to feel anxious while waiting for changes to happen, or to worry about side effects. Having realistic time frames and honest talks with the doctor can lower unnecessary stress.

If side effects occur, it is best to speak with a professional rather than just quitting suddenly. Some side effects subside over time, while others might need a dosage adjustment or a switch in treatment.

10.18 Combining Medical and Non-Medical Approaches

Many doctors suggest that men continue using gentle hair care routines, manage stress, and maintain good nutrition while on medical treatments. For example, a man might be on finasteride, use a mild shampoo, follow a healthy diet, and try scalp massages a couple of times a week. This multi-angle approach can support the best possible environment for hair.

10.19 Common Questions About Medical Treatments

1. **When Should I Start?**
   Some men begin as soon as they see a receding hairline or thinning areas, believing early action slows future loss. Others wait until hair loss is more noticeable. There is no single perfect moment, but starting sooner can help preserve existing hair.
2. **How Long Until I See Results?**
   Oral medications like finasteride often take 3-6 months to show changes. Minoxidil can also need several months. Transplant results become clear after 6-12 months, as hair goes through natural growth cycles.
3. **Are These Treatments Safe?**
   Millions of men use finasteride and minoxidil. They are generally safe, but side effects are possible. Surgery has standard surgical risks like infection or scarring. A qualified doctor can reduce these chances.
4. **Do I Need Blood Tests?**
   Sometimes, yes—especially if the doctor suspects a thyroid or hormone imbalance.

Chapter 11: Hair Care Methods for Healthier Strands)

Most people think of hair care as simple: just shampoo, rinse, and go. But many small details can come together to make hair look stronger, shinier, and fuller. This is especially helpful for men dealing with thinning or shedding. Proper hair care can't always stop genetic issues, but it can protect the strands you still have, slow breakage, and create an overall healthier scalp environment.

In this chapter, we will explore a range of hair care methods suited for men. We will look at the benefits of certain products, best practices for washing and styling, and ways to limit day-to-day damage. While these steps may seem basic, sticking to them consistently can pay off over the long run—especially if thinning or weak hair is a concern.

11.1 Foundations of Hair Care

11.1.1 Why It Matters

If someone has inherited genes for hair loss or faces hormonal factors, they might wonder how important hair care really is. After all, if the follicles are going to shrink from DHT, does washing or styling matter? The reality is, hair care can't change genetic or hormone-driven thinning, but it can protect the hair that is still growing. Also, caring for the scalp is key. A balanced, clean scalp is less likely to suffer from itchiness, inflammation, or buildup that might speed up shedding.

11.1.2 Common Mistakes

Many men wash their hair too roughly or too often with harsh shampoos, assume a quick rinse is enough, or use styling methods that tug or break strands. Another frequent mistake is skipping conditioner, thinking it's "for women" or only for people with very long hair. But men's hair can benefit from conditioner too, particularly if it's getting thin or brittle.

11.2 Choosing the Right Products

11.2.1 Shampoos

Shampoo removes dirt, oils, and dead skin cells. But some shampoos may be too harsh, leading to dryness or irritation over time.

1. **Gentle vs. Harsh Ingredients:** Look for shampoos without high levels of sulfates (like sodium lauryl sulfate). Sulfates foam well but can also strip too much oil from the scalp.
2. **pH Balance:** A pH-balanced shampoo is less likely to leave hair strands rough or the scalp overly dry.
3. **Frequency:** Men with oily scalps might wash daily or every other day, while those with drier scalps might do so 2-3 times a week. Adjust based on how your hair and scalp feel.

11.2.2 Conditioners

Conditioner coats the outside of the hair shaft and helps seal the cuticle layer. A sealed cuticle reduces friction and prevents split ends.

1. **Types of Conditioner:**
   - **Daily Rinse-Out:** Applied to wet hair after shampooing, left for a minute or so, then rinsed.
   - **Deep Conditioner or Mask:** Left on for longer (5-20 minutes) to provide more moisture or repair.
2. **Protein-Based Conditioners:** Can strengthen weak hair shafts. Be aware that too much protein might cause stiffness if hair is already well-proteinated, so balance is key.
3. **Leave-In Conditioners:** Light sprays or creams that remain in the hair. Helpful for detangling or adding some volume, especially in thinner hair.

11.2.3 Specialized Products

- **Anti-Dandruff Shampoos:** If you have flaking or itching, products with zinc pyrithione, salicylic acid, or other active ingredients might help.

- **Volumizing Shampoos and Conditioners:** Formulated to add temporary fullness, often by coating hair fibers or reducing excess oils that weigh hair down.
- **Clarifying Shampoos:** Remove heavy buildup from styling products, though they shouldn't be used too often as they can be drying.

11.3 Washing Methods and Best Practices

11.3.1 Wetting the Hair Thoroughly

Soaking your hair completely for several seconds before applying shampoo helps create a better lather with less product. This cuts down on the risk of scrubbing the scalp too aggressively just to get the shampoo evenly distributed.

11.3.2 Amount of Shampoo

Men often use more shampoo than needed. Usually, a nickel- or quarter-sized amount (depending on hair length and thickness) suffices. Rubbing shampoo between your hands before applying helps spread it more evenly.

11.3.3 Gentle Massage Technique

Use your fingertips, not your nails, to massage the scalp. This removes dirt and oil while boosting blood flow. Harsh scrubbing can irritate follicles. In thinning areas, be especially gentle to avoid dislodging weak hairs.

11.3.4 Rinse Thoroughly

Leftover shampoo or conditioner can weigh hair down or lead to scalp irritation. Taking an extra few seconds to rinse fully can make a noticeable difference in how hair looks and feels.

11.3.5 Temperature of Water

Many men like hot showers, but very hot water can dry the scalp and possibly worsen breakage. Lukewarm or moderately warm water is often best. Some stylists suggest a cool rinse at the end to help close hair cuticles, though the effect can be modest.

11.4 Drying and Towel Techniques

11.4.1 Avoid Vigorously Rubbing

When stepping out of the shower, hair is more fragile because the cuticle layer is open. Rough towel-rubbing can stretch and snap wet strands. A better approach is to gently pat or squeeze out the excess moisture.

11.4.2 Air Dry vs. Blow Dry

- **Air Dry:** Letting hair air dry is the gentlest option in most cases. However, men who prefer a certain style or need quick drying might use a blow dryer.
- **Blow Dry:** To reduce heat damage, use the dryer on a lower setting and hold it a few inches away from the scalp. Moving the dryer around, rather than focusing on one spot, can prevent overheating.
- **Heat Protectants:** Some light sprays or creams can lessen the harm from heat styling, though men don't always think to use them.

11.4.3 Comb When Partially Dry

Comb or brush hair when it's partially dry, not dripping wet, to reduce tension on the strands. Wide-toothed combs or soft-bristle brushes are helpful for preventing tangles in longer styles.

11.5 Styling Wisely

11.5.1 Type of Styling Products

1. **Gels:** Offer strong hold but can leave the hair stiff or sticky. Some gels contain alcohol, which might dry out the scalp if used frequently.

2. **Pomades or Waxes:** Good for a slick look or to add texture. However, heavy pomades might block the scalp if not washed out thoroughly.
3. **Creams or Pastes:** Provide moderate hold without the stiffness of gels. They can help add slight volume to thinner hair.
4. **Hairsprays:** Useful for setting a style in place, though some contain chemicals that might irritate sensitive scalps over time.

11.5.2 Avoid Overapplication

Using too much product can weigh hair down and make thinning areas more obvious. Start with a small amount and add more only if needed. Washing out styling products fully at the end of the day reduces buildup.

11.5.3 Gentle Techniques

Pulling hair tight or creating severe styles might put stress on follicles. While many men don't often wear tight braids, even a pulled-back man bun can strain hair if done forcefully each day. Rotating styles or giving the scalp breaks can help.

11.6 Dealing with Different Hair Types

11.6.1 Fine Hair

Men with fine hair might find it looks limp or easily weighed down by products. Lightweight shampoos and conditioners, plus minimal styling product, can help keep fine strands from going flat. A volumizing mousse can add some lift.

11.6.2 Curly or Wavy Hair

Curly hair can tangle more easily and might appear frizzy if not moisturized properly. A leave-in conditioner can help control frizz. It's also better to avoid excessive brushing of curly hair, as it can break the shape of the curl and lead to bigger tangles.

11.6.3 Coarse or Thick Hair

Coarse hair may need more moisture to remain flexible and manageable. Deep conditioning treatments once a week can keep strands from getting rough or overly dry. Men with thick hair should also be mindful of scalp buildup, ensuring shampoo reaches the skin rather than just the outer hair layer.

11.7 Scalp Care

11.7.1 Recognizing Scalp Problems

Common issues like dandruff (flakes), dryness, or mild psoriasis can all affect hair health. An irritated scalp might result in extra shedding. Some helpful tips:

- **Excess Oil:** If the scalp seems greasy, use a clarifying or balancing shampoo.
- **Flaking and Itching:** Shampoos with zinc pyrithione, salicylic acid, or selenium sulfide can reduce flakes.
- **Redness or Burning:** Seek advice from a medical professional, as stronger treatments may be necessary if there's infection or persistent inflammation.

11.7.2 Massages and Circulation

A gentle scalp massage once or twice a week can boost blood flow. Use the pads of your fingers in small circular motions. Some men add a bit of natural oil like jojoba or sweet almond oil for extra comfort. This doesn't guarantee new hair growth but can keep the scalp pliable and less tense.

11.8 External Factors to Watch

11.8.1 Sun Exposure

Men with thinning hair have less protection on the scalp. Extended sun exposure can result in burns, dryness, or peeling. Wearing a hat (not too tight) or applying sunscreen lotion designed for the scalp can help. There are spray sunscreens made especially for thinning hair, which go on lightly.

11.8.2 Chlorine and Salt Water

Chlorine in pools and salt in the ocean can dry out the hair shaft. Rinsing hair with fresh water soon after swimming reduces the chance of dryness or brittle strands. Some men use a protective leave-in conditioner before swimming as well.

11.8.3 Pollution and Dust

Living in a highly polluted area can mean dust and grime settle on the scalp regularly. More frequent gentle washing or using a mild clarifying product can combat this buildup without stripping essential oils.

11.9 Tools for Better Hair Care

11.9.1 Wide-Toothed Combs

Great for detangling without too much pulling. Plastic combs with smooth, rounded teeth can be kinder to the scalp.

11.9.2 Boar-Bristle Brushes

These brushes distribute natural oils from the scalp through the hair. However, they are usually more useful for men with medium to long hair. If you have very short hair, a soft-bristle brush might do.

11.9.3 Microfiber Towels

Regular cotton towels can be rough. Microfiber towels absorb water more efficiently and create less friction, which can help reduce breakage after washing.

11.10 Occasional Deep Treatments

11.10.1 Deep Conditioning or Hair Masks

Applying a richer formula once every week or two can give a boost of moisture and nutrients to dry or stressed hair. Ingredients like shea butter, argan oil, or keratin can help fill minor gaps in damaged cuticles.

11.10.2 Protein Treatments

These can temporarily fortify hair strands. For those with hair breakage, a protein treatment can be done monthly or every few weeks. Overuse might lead to stiff, crunchy hair, so it's best not to do it too often.

11.10.3 Scalp Scrubs or Peels

Some brands sell gentle scalp scrubs to lift dead skin or leftover products. Use these cautiously—once a month or so—and pick those with mild exfoliants. Excessive scrubbing can inflame the scalp.

11.11 Handling Damage from Styling Tools

11.11.1 Heat Styling Precautions

Men who straighten hair or frequently blow-dry on high heat might notice dryness or split ends. Using a heat protectant spray or serum can form a barrier. Lowering the temperature setting on styling tools helps as well.

11.11.2 Chemical Services

Men who bleach or dye their hair need to be aware that chemicals can weaken the hair shaft. Spacing out such procedures and following them with nourishing treatments can prevent extensive harm.

11.11.3 Regular Trims

Trimming off split ends can make hair look healthier, even if it doesn't increase the quantity of hair on the scalp. It also stops splits from creeping up the shaft.

11.12 Nighttime Hair Care

11.12.1 Sleeping Postures

If hair is long enough to get tangled, men might tie it loosely or use a satin pillowcase to reduce friction. A very tight ponytail or bun at night can stress follicles, so avoid tension.

11.12.2 Overnight Treatments

Some hair oils or leave-in conditioners are meant to be used overnight. They can help with dryness, but be sure to wash or partially rinse in the morning if the formula is heavy, to avoid buildup.

11.13 When to Seek Expert Help

Sometimes hair issues are bigger than dryness or mild breakage. If you notice sudden, large amounts of shedding, big bald patches, constant itching, or scalp sores, it's wise to see a professional. A dermatologist or a trichologist can check if there's a deeper scalp disorder or an infection.

11.14 Lifestyle Overlaps

Healthy hair care does not end in the bathroom. What you eat, how you handle stress, and whether you get enough sleep all support or weaken hair health. For example:

- **Nutrition:** Lack of protein, vitamins, or minerals can cause hair to look dull or break.
- **Stress:** High stress can show up in the hair cycle. Good self-care might reduce shedding.
- **Exercise:** Moderate exercise boosts circulation, which can help deliver nutrients to the scalp.

Keeping an eye on these external factors while practicing smart hair care can amplify the results.

11.15 Common Misconceptions

1. **Daily Shampooing is Always Bad:** Not necessarily. It depends on scalp oil production and the type of shampoo. Some men produce more oil and do fine washing daily.
2. **You Shouldn't Use Conditioner if You Have Short Hair:** Short hair can still benefit from moisture and protection.
3. **Hair Care Doesn't Matter if You're Going Bald Anyway:** Even if genetic hair loss is present, caring for your existing hair can keep it looking healthier and might slow breakage-based thinning.

11.16 A Sample Hair Care Routine

While everyone's hair is different, here's a simple example routine for an average man with mild thinning:

1. **Morning:**

- Shower with a mild shampoo 3-4 times a week, especially if scalp gets oily.
- Use a light conditioner each time you shampoo. Rinse well.
- Pat hair dry with a microfiber towel.
- Apply a small amount of styling cream if desired.

2. **Evening:**
    - If using products during the day, rinse scalp lightly to clear any buildup.
    - Twice a week, apply a scalp massage with a small amount of natural oil for a few minutes.
    - If hair is long enough, tie it loosely or just leave it free when sleeping.
3. **Weekly or Bi-weekly Extras:**
    - Use a deep conditioning mask or protein treatment to strengthen hair.
    - Switch to a clarifying shampoo once every two weeks if using many styling products.

This is just a guide. Adjust based on your hair's texture, length, and how it responds.

11.17 Consistency is Key

The biggest part of effective hair care is doing it regularly. A single deep conditioning session once a year or an occasional gentle shampoo won't do much if the rest of the time hair is handled poorly. Small steps add up over weeks and months, helping hair look its best and reducing the impact of natural shedding.

Chapter 12: Surgical Procedures and Their Outcomes

For men who have already experienced significant thinning or complete loss in some areas, everyday hair care or medications might not restore the look of a full head of hair. In such cases, surgical procedures can offer a more permanent result. While these approaches involve cost, time, and some level of risk, they may provide a real change for those wanting to rebuild a hairline or fill in large bald spots.

This chapter discusses the primary surgical methods available for hair loss, focusing on hair transplant techniques and some newer or less common procedures. We will cover how these surgeries work, who they are best suited for, what results can be expected, and what risks men should be aware of before choosing them.

12.1 Why Surgery for Hair Loss?

Surgical options often appeal to men whose hair loss has progressed beyond what medications or non-medical fixes can handle. Men who see very thin or bald zones, especially around the front or crown, might find that topical or oral treatments only slow further loss rather than restoring lost hair. Surgery aims to physically move healthy hairs into these areas or otherwise alter the scalp in ways that make hair appear thicker.

Major reasons to consider surgical procedures:

- **Permanent Results:** Unlike medications that must be continued indefinitely, a successful hair transplant can last many years, as transplanted hair usually stays put if done correctly.
- **Advanced Hair Loss:** Men in late stages of pattern baldness might not get enough coverage from topical or oral treatments alone.
- **Control Over Hairline Design:** A transplant can restore a more youthful hairline, which can boost a person's confidence if a receding line was a source of distress.

12.2 Hair Transplant Basics

A hair transplant, in simple terms, moves hair follicles from a donor site—usually the back or sides of the scalp—to thinning or bald zones (recipient site). The reason donor hair is taken from these regions is because the follicles there are often more resistant to DHT, meaning they keep growing even if placed in a hair loss-prone area on top.

12.2.1 Two Main Methods: FUT and FUE

1. **FUT (Follicular Unit Transplantation):**
    - **Process:** A surgeon removes a strip of scalp from the back (donor area). The strip is then dissected into small grafts containing 1 to 4 hair follicles each. These grafts are placed into tiny incisions in the recipient site.
    - **Pros:** Allows many grafts to be harvested in a single session. Often more cost-effective.
    - **Cons:** Leaves a linear scar where the strip was taken. Recovery can be longer or slightly more uncomfortable.
2. **FUE (Follicular Unit Extraction):**
    - **Process:** Instead of removing a strip, the surgeon extracts individual follicles with a tiny punch. Each follicular unit is then transplanted similarly into the balding area.
    - **Pros:** No linear scar, often a quicker healing time. Potentially less scarring if done well.
    - **Cons:** Can be time-consuming for large sessions, may be more expensive. Requires a skilled practitioner to avoid damage to follicles during extraction.

12.2.2 Steps Involved

1. **Consultation:** The surgeon checks the scalp, donor area, and hair loss pattern. They discuss goals and whether the patient's expectations are realistic.
2. **Pre-Op Preparation:** Patients might be asked to avoid certain medications or alcohol. They might need to stop smoking if they do, as smoking can slow healing.

3. **Anesthesia:** Hair transplant procedures are typically performed under local anesthesia. The patient is awake but does not feel pain in the scalp.
4. **Harvesting Donor Hair:** Either the strip (FUT) or individual follicles (FUE) are taken.
5. **Graft Preparation:** Technicians separate the grafts into groups of 1-4 hairs each (follicular units).
6. **Recipient Site Incisions:** Small slits or holes are made in the balding area at angles that mimic natural hair growth.
7. **Placing the Grafts:** Each graft is carefully inserted, aiming for a natural look.
8. **Post-Op Care:** The scalp may be bandaged, and patients receive care instructions to prevent infection or dislodging of grafts.

12.3 Recovery and Aftercare

12.3.1 Immediate Post-Op

- **Scab Formation:** Small scabs often form around each implanted graft. They usually fall off within a week or two.
- **Swelling:** Some patients have mild swelling in the forehead or around the donor area, which typically fades in a few days.
- **Pain Management:** There may be some discomfort, especially with the FUT method due to the linear scar. Pain relievers can help.

12.3.2 Shedding the Transplanted Hair

A common surprise is that the newly transplanted hairs often fall out within 2-4 weeks. This is normal. The follicle remains in the scalp, but the shaft is shed as the follicle resets to a new growth cycle. Actual regrowth typically starts around 3-4 months after surgery.

12.3.3 Long-Term Results

By around 8-12 months post-operation, patients see the final outcome: new hair that grows, can be cut or styled, and typically behaves like hair from the donor region. This hair is often more stable against future DHT effects, but men must remember the surrounding, non-transplanted hair can still thin over time without proper care or medical treatments.

12.4 Who Qualifies for a Hair Transplant?

Not everyone is a perfect candidate. Surgeons consider:

1. **Age:** Usually, it's best to wait until at least mid-20s or later, when hair loss patterns are clearer.
2. **Extent of Hair Loss:** The more donor hair available and the smaller the recipient area, the better the outcome might be.
3. **Donor Area Quality:** Thick hair on the back or sides of the head provides better grafts. Men with very sparse donor regions may not achieve the coverage they want.
4. **Health:** Conditions like uncontrolled diabetes or bleeding disorders can complicate surgery or healing. Smoking also slows recovery.
5. **Realistic Expectations:** Those who expect an unrealistic level of fullness might be disappointed. Surgeons often explain what is possible with the available donor hair.

12.5 Potential Risks and Complications

All surgeries carry some risk. While hair transplants are generally safe, a few complications include:

1. **Infection:** Rare, but possible. Proper sterile techniques and aftercare reduce this risk.
2. **Bleeding or Scarring:** FUT leaves a linear scar; FUE can leave small round scars if not done properly.
3. **Shock Loss:** Sometimes existing hairs near the transplant area can temporarily shed due to stress on the scalp. They often regrow.
4. **Poor Graft Survival:** If not enough grafts survive, the result can look patchy. Skilled surgeons take care to maximize survival rate.

5. **Unnatural Hairline:** If angles or placement are done poorly, the hairline can appear fake or obviously transplanted.

Choosing a reputable, experienced surgeon greatly lowers the chance of these problems. It's crucial to ask for before-and-after photos of previous patients, read reviews, and possibly get multiple opinions.

12.6 Cost and Time Considerations

Hair transplant costs vary widely based on region, surgeon expertise, and the number of grafts needed. It can range from a few thousand to tens of thousands of dollars. Some men opt for clinics in other countries where prices are lower, but quality can also vary. Doing thorough research is key.

Time-wise, a single session can last from 4-8 hours or more, depending on how many grafts are transplanted. A large area of baldness might need multiple sessions spaced months apart for best results.

12.7 Other Surgical Methods

12.7.1 Scalp Reduction

An older procedure less common now, scalp reduction removes bald areas of the scalp surgically and pulls together the remaining parts that still have hair. This can reduce the size of a bald patch, but it may create visible scarring or a "stretch-back" effect. Medications or hair transplants often replaced scalp reductions for cosmetic reasons.

12.7.2 Flap Surgery

Involves moving a flap of scalp with healthy hair to a balding area. This is an even less common approach today due to complexity and risk of unnatural growth directions. It also can lead to scarring along the flap edges.

12.7.3 Hairline Lowering (Forehead Reduction)

For some individuals, this is done to reduce a high forehead. Surgeons remove a small area of forehead skin and pull the hair-bearing scalp forward. It's more of a cosmetic fix for forehead proportion rather than classic hair loss, though some men do it to address receding hairlines if they also have a naturally high hairline.

12.8 Combining Surgery with Other Treatments

Many men who opt for a transplant also continue using finasteride or minoxidil. These medications help preserve the hair they already have, reducing further thinning. Combining both surgical and medical approaches can maintain an overall fuller look. Without ongoing treatment, the native hair (non-transplanted) might keep thinning around the transplanted grafts, leading to patchy patterns in the future.

12.9 Scalp Micropigmentation (SMP) and Surgery

Scalp micropigmentation can be used on its own or alongside a transplant. For example:

- **Filling Gaps:** After a transplant, some men use SMP to add the illusion of thicker density between grafts.
- **Covering Scars:** SMP can camouflage the linear scar from FUT or small round scars from FUE. This is done by tattooing small dots that match hair color.

12.10 Realistic Outcomes

While hair transplant surgeries can achieve impressive transformations, they rarely produce the same hair density a man had as a teenager. A successful result often looks natural but may still appear thinner than a fully thick scalp. Skilled surgeons know how to place grafts for the best visual effect, using a blend of single-hair grafts at the hairline and multi-hair grafts behind that zone to add bulk.

12.11 Personal Stories and Scenarios

1. **Case A:** A man in his early 30s with a receding hairline. He has a strong donor area and decides on FUE to fill in the frontal zone. After healing, he continues finasteride to protect the rest of his hair. By one year post-op, he sees a fuller hairline that looks natural.
2. **Case B:** Another man in his 40s with a large bald crown. He opts for FUT to get a bigger number of grafts in one go. While the linear scar is present, he keeps the back hair slightly long to hide it. He's happy with the coverage but knows he might need a second session for more density.
3. **Case C:** A patient with limited donor hair who tries a small FUE session but the results aren't enough to cover his entire scalp. He then chooses scalp micropigmentation to add the look of thickness around the transplanted hair. The combined effect is subtle but better than before.

12.12 Preparing Mentally and Practically

Men considering surgery should keep in mind:

- **Healing Time:** Plan for at least a few days to a week of taking it easy, especially if your job is physical. The scalp might look red or have scabs for up to two weeks.
- **Hair Shedding Phase:** Don't panic when transplanted hairs fall out in the first month. That's normal, and new hairs generally grow in later.
- **Setting Realistic Goals:** Talk with the surgeon about how many grafts are needed, how many sessions might be required, and the best approach for your unique situation.

- **Avoiding Unqualified Providers:** Bargain deals might be tempting, but poor surgical work can be hard to fix and may lead to permanent scarring.

12.13 Follow-Up Sessions

Sometimes a single surgery can achieve a patient's goals, but many need multiple sessions. For example, the patient might restore the front hairline in one session, then address the crown in a future procedure. If hair loss continues over the years, additional touch-ups might be planned. Consistent check-ins with a hair specialist can track changes and decide if more grafts are needed.

12.14 Special Considerations

1. **Younger Men:** Those in their early 20s might still have a changing hair loss pattern. Surgeons sometimes suggest waiting until it's clearer how it will progress.
2. **Patients with Scarring Alopecia:** They might have areas of scar tissue that affect graft survival. Special methods or a test patch might be needed.
3. **Ethnic Differences:** Different hair types (curly, coarse, or fine) can affect how a transplant is done and how a hairline is shaped for a natural look.
4. **Women:** Though this book focuses on men, note that some women also get hair transplant surgeries. The basics are similar, but hairline shaping may differ.

12.15 Future Trends in Surgical Procedures

Research continues to improve hair transplant technology:

- **Robotic FUE Systems:** Machines can assist surgeons in extracting follicles more precisely. Some clinics use robotic arms that identify and punch out grafts with minimal damage.

- **Improved Graft Storage Solutions:** Keeping grafts in specialized growth factor solutions might boost survival rates once transplanted.
- **Hair Cloning or Tissue Engineering:** Still experimental. Could eventually provide an unlimited donor supply if scientists can grow new follicles from a patient's own cells.

12.16 Balancing Cost, Benefit, and Expectations

Before committing to surgery, men must weigh:

- **Cost:** Is the final outcome worth the financial investment?
- **Time and Healing:** Can you take time off for the procedure and recover properly?
- **Realistic Gains:** Does a partial improvement (rather than a fully dense scalp) still meet your goals?
- **Long-Term Maintenance:** Are you willing to stay on medication or possibly plan for more surgeries if hair loss progresses?

Speaking openly with the surgical team helps clarify these points. A second opinion can also be wise if you're unsure about the recommended plan.

12.17 Non-Surgical Alternatives for Significant Loss

If someone has very limited donor hair, or if they can't afford surgery, there are still ways to improve appearance:

- **Hair Systems (Wigs/Toppers):** Modern options can be quite realistic.
- **Scalp Micropigmentation:** Gives the look of shaved or thicker hair.
- **Lifestyle and Cosmetic Measures:** Using hair fibers or a suitable style.

Surgery isn't the only path. It's an option that gives permanent results but does come with certain demands and expenses.

Chapter 13: Future Trends in Hair Loss Solutions

Efforts to address hair loss have been around for centuries, with many attempts that range from folklore remedies to modern science. Today, research continues to uncover new ways to understand and possibly solve hair thinning in men. These developments include high-tech devices, advanced medical compounds, and even potential breakthroughs in growing new hair follicles in laboratories. While some of these approaches are in early stages, they offer a glimpse of how the field might change in the coming years.

In this chapter, we will explore various future trends and ongoing research that may lead to more advanced solutions for hair loss. Some of these might be widely available soon, while others remain experimental. Although there are no firm guarantees, keeping informed about these trends can help men prepare for promising options and discuss them with experts when the time is right.

13.1 Current Gaps in Hair Loss Treatments

Before delving into future ideas, it helps to note why new solutions are needed in the first place. Many existing treatments—like finasteride, minoxidil, or hair transplant surgery—can be quite helpful. However, they have certain limits:

1. **Partial Response:** Some men do not respond well to current medications. Finasteride may slow hair loss for many users, but it might not produce enough visible regrowth. Minoxidil can thicken existing hair, yet it rarely brings back large areas of lost hair.
2. **Lifetime Use:** Stopping these treatments often leads to a return of hair loss symptoms. This can be expensive and inconvenient over decades.
3. **Side Effects or Risks:** Finasteride, dutasteride, and other hormone-targeting drugs can carry possible side effects. Some men

avoid or discontinue these because they feel the risks outweigh the benefits.
4. **Surgery Challenges:** Hair transplants offer a more enduring fix, but they're costly, require surgical skill, and depend on having a good donor area. Some men simply do not qualify or cannot afford them.

These gaps fuel scientists to seek more efficient, long-lasting, and safer approaches.

13.2 Advances in Topical and Oral Medications

13.2.1 New Formulations of Existing Drugs

Many researchers are looking at ways to refine existing medications to reduce side effects and improve results. For instance, newer topical finasteride formulas aim to keep the drug's action mostly in the scalp, lowering the amount that enters the bloodstream. This could help men who avoid oral finasteride due to potential systemic effects.

There are also tests to combine minoxidil with other compounds that enhance scalp absorption, so that the product can penetrate deeper. This might mean people need less frequent applications or see quicker results. While these advances are not as dramatic as an entirely new drug, they may still make the experience of using known treatments more pleasant and reliable.

13.2.2 Cutting-Edge Molecules

Along with refining existing drugs, new molecules that target different parts of the hair growth process are being studied. Researchers might zero in on:

- **Stem Cells in Follicles:** Some compounds attempt to stimulate or protect these crucial cells.
- **Growth Factor Manipulation:** Certain natural proteins in the body can spur hair growth. If these can be delivered directly to follicles, hair might grow better.

- **Anti-Inflammatory Agents:** Since inflammation can harm follicles, specialized anti-inflammatory molecules may extend the active growth phase.

In some cases, these compounds have shown promise in lab studies on animals or in small human trials, but more testing is needed before they reach everyday clinics.

13.3 Gene Therapy Possibilities

13.3.1 Understanding Genetic Triggers

We have already learned that genes play a large role in male pattern hair loss. Scientists keep searching for the specific genes or gene combinations that decide how follicles respond to hormones like DHT. If these can be pinpointed, gene therapy might allow doctors to switch off or mute harmful genetic signals.

13.3.2 Methods of Gene Editing

New tools such as CRISPR have made gene editing more accessible in theory, but applying these methods safely to humans is complex. In theory, one could inject a gene-editing compound that targets hair follicles to:

- Lower DHT sensitivity.
- Boost hair cell regeneration.
- Activate dormant follicles.

Still, the technology faces major hurdles, including safety, targeted delivery, and ethical considerations. Altering genes in a way that affects the entire body is risky, so efforts focus on localized or temporary editing in scalp tissues. It may be many years before this becomes a routine option—if it ever does.

13.4 Hair Cloning and Regenerative Techniques

13.4.1 Lab-Grown Follicles

One of the most discussed future ideas is hair cloning, sometimes called "follicle multiplication." Scientists want to extract a small sample of a person's healthy follicles, replicate them in a lab, and then implant these new follicles back into the scalp. If successful, this could give an unlimited supply of donor hair—solving the biggest problem faced in hair transplants (the limited donor region).

Key challenges include:

- **Keeping Follicles Stable:** Follicles grown in labs can lose their structure or function over time.
- **Positioning:** Once implanted, the new follicles must align correctly in the scalp and continue normal hair cycling.
- **Scarring or Rejection:** The body might not always accept lab-grown tissues, although using the patient's own cells should reduce rejection risks.

A few clinics and biotech firms are actively trying to push this technology forward. Some have announced partial successes in growing follicle-like structures, but large-scale human trials are still needed to confirm lasting results.

13.4.2 Stem Cell Therapies

Stem cells are unique because they can develop into various cell types, including hair follicle cells. Scientists are looking at ways to gather stem cells from fat, blood, or bone marrow, then inject them into the scalp to spur hair regeneration. Some clinics offer "stem cell injections," but their processes vary a lot, and many are not yet proven with strong, peer-reviewed studies.

If a more controlled approach arises—where a man's own stem cells are refined and directed to become fully functioning follicle units—it could transform hair loss treatment. However, this is still in development and may require many steps, like laboratory growth of cells, specialized injection methods, and follow-up care.

13.5 Smart Delivery Systems

Even current medications might work better if scientists perfect delivery to the follicle. Some labs are testing "nano-carriers" or "microcapsules" that transport drugs right to the hair root. This could mean:

- Lower doses, reducing systemic side effects.
- More consistent results by ensuring each follicle gets enough medication.
- Controlled release over days or weeks, so users do not need to apply something daily.

Such systems might help men who forget to apply treatments or who dislike daily routines. They might also cut costs by reducing wasted product. But it's important that the materials in these carriers do not irritate the skin or get stuck in the scalp's pores. Research in this area is ongoing.

13.6 Low-Level Laser and Light Advancements

Laser therapy has been around for a while, but there's growing interest in more advanced devices. Scientists are investigating whether different light wavelengths or pulse patterns can better stimulate follicles. Some devices combine laser light with other energy sources, like ultrasound, in an attempt to accelerate results.

Future devices might:

- Adjust automatically to the user's scalp condition.
- Track hair density changes over time and modify settings accordingly.
- Sync with apps or cloud-based platforms for personalized schedules.

Though these ideas remain theoretical, technology moves quickly. If these advanced machines are proven effective, they could turn into new home or clinic-based options for men who prefer non-invasive methods.

13.7 Microbiome Research on the Scalp

Your scalp, like your gut or skin, hosts billions of microbes (bacteria, fungi, etc.). Scientists have started investigating the "scalp microbiome" to see if certain microbial imbalances might worsen hair loss or scalp inflammation. Early findings suggest that some microorganisms could protect follicles, while others irritate the scalp.

In the future, specialized shampoos or scalp treatments might be designed to restore a healthy microbial balance. By feeding or introducing beneficial microbes, or reducing harmful ones, it might be possible to create an ideal environment for hair to thrive. This approach is still quite new, but it reflects a larger trend in medicine—focusing on balancing natural communities of microbes rather than just killing them.

13.8 Hormone and Receptor Blocking Innovations

We know that male pattern hair loss is closely linked to DHT. Blocking DHT systemically (like with finasteride) can help, but also affects the entire body. Researchers are exploring molecules that block DHT or androgen receptors purely in the scalp. If that works well, men might see:

- **Fewer Sexual Side Effects:** Because hormone levels in other parts of the body remain normal.
- **Stronger Local Impact:** More hair preservation in affected areas.
- **Fewer Daily Steps:** Possibly a longer-acting injection or implant that blocks receptors for months.

Any method that localizes the effect must do so without irritating the scalp or losing potency quickly. Achieving this balance is tricky, but the possibility could transform the way men treat androgen-related hair loss.

13.9 Artificial Intelligence in Diagnosis and Personalized Plans

13.9.1 Scalp Imaging and Analysis

Artificial intelligence (AI) has entered many health fields. One emerging idea is using AI-based imaging devices to scan the scalp, count hairs, and measure thickness automatically. This can detect early changes that might be invisible to the naked eye. Over time, AI could:

- Monitor a user's progress on certain treatments.
- Compare results with a large database of men with similar hair types and patterns.
- Recommend small modifications (like adjusting topical dosage) based on real-time scalp data.

13.9.2 Personalized Advice

Additionally, AI might help generate custom hair loss plans. By factoring in a person's genetics, lifestyle, stress levels, and scalp health, an advanced algorithm could suggest the best combination of medications, scalp therapies, or nutritional changes. This would move beyond the "one-size-fits-all" approach many men use now, potentially increasing success rates.

13.10 Longer-Lasting Solutions and Implants

Some research is focused on synthetic hair implants, though these have been tried in the past with limited success. Newer materials aim to be more biocompatible, reducing the risk of inflammation and rejection. If perfected, synthetic implants could let men achieve a desired hair density without needing donor hair. However, the challenge is ensuring these implants look natural, stay in place, and do not harm the scalp over time.

There is also the possibility of micro-implants that slowly release growth factors or medications directly into the scalp. Similar to how certain birth control implants work in the arm, a device could be placed beneath the skin to consistently drip helpful substances around follicles. But any foreign object placed under the skin risks infection or other complications, so careful design and trial data are needed.

13.11 Integrative Approaches

Another trend is integrative or "holistic" approaches that combine scientific treatments with broader lifestyle and wellness measures in a single plan. A clinic might bring together specialists in dermatology, nutrition, stress management, and even mental health to address hair loss from multiple angles. This is partly an extension of current advice (eat well, reduce stress, treat scalp problems) but with more structured programs and monitoring.

Some advanced clinics may offer:

- **On-site blood tests** to check hormone and nutrient levels.
- **Genetic and TrichoTest results** to tailor medication choices.
- **Scalp health sessions** with specialized devices for cleansing, light therapy, or gentle chemical peels.
- **Lifestyle coaching** to maintain consistent sleep, exercise, and diet routines.

Though these integrative centers can be expensive, they might become more common if results prove better than using single treatments alone.

13.12 Regulatory Hurdles and Timelines

It is important to remember that bringing new hair loss solutions to the market involves regulation by health authorities. Any new drug or device must go through clinical trials, which can take years. This process ensures safety and effectiveness but also slows availability.

When you read headlines about "new hair growth breakthroughs," it can be tempting to think a cure is just around the corner. Often, these stories highlight early-phase research in mice or small human trials. There could be many steps left—larger trials, approval, manufacturing, and distribution. Some promising ideas fade away if they fail in advanced testing.

13.13 Potential Ethical and Social Questions

If hair cloning or gene therapy for hair loss becomes real, there may be concerns:

- **Access and Cost:** Will only wealthy individuals be able to afford these advanced procedures, widening a gap in cosmetic appearance between different income levels?
- **Long-Term Effects:** Gene editing or cloned follicles might have unknown risks decades later.
- **Pressure to Look "Perfect":** As solutions improve, some men might feel more forced to treat any sign of thinning, rather than accept a natural process.

Balancing these concerns with individual freedom to choose treatments will be an ongoing debate. Regulators, medical bodies, and the public will need to discuss how to handle these breakthroughs responsibly.

13.14 What Men Can Do Now to Stay Updated

1. **Consult Knowledgeable Professionals:** Dermatologists and hair restoration doctors often keep track of new studies and can share realistic updates.
2. **Attend Hair Loss Conferences or Webinars:** Some events are open to the public and feature experts discussing the latest research.
3. **Join Patient Groups or Forums:** While these can sometimes spread hype, they can also provide early news about clinical trials or personal experiences.
4. **Read Peer-Reviewed Articles:** Scientific journals or reputable news outlets covering medical research can provide a clearer picture of what is real and what is still unproven.

13.15 Trying Experimental Treatments: Risks and Rewards

Some men volunteer for clinical trials or try "off-label" uses of new therapies. This can give them early access to cutting-edge methods, but also carries uncertainty. It is important to:

- **Fully Understand the Trial Protocol:** Know the possible risks, side effects, and time commitment.
- **Confirm the Credibility of the Clinic or Study:** Avoid unregulated, shady offers that claim breakthroughs without any data.
- **Discuss with a Doctor:** A trusted physician can help weigh pros and cons.

While volunteering may feel like a leap of faith, it also helps advance science, potentially benefiting future men with hair loss.

13.16 A Glimpse of Tomorrow

Some experts imagine a future where men could walk into a clinic, have a small patch of scalp biopsied, and within a few weeks or months, an unlimited supply of healthy follicle cells would be ready for transplantation. Or, with gene therapy, a single injection might "switch off" DHT sensitivity in scalp follicles. These scenarios might seem like science fiction today, but they reflect real lines of research. How quickly they become standard practice depends on success rates, safety data, and acceptance by the medical community.

13.17 Staying Grounded

Even as we anticipate these exciting possibilities, it is wise to remain grounded. Breakthroughs sometimes take much longer than expected, or they arrive but only partially solve the problem. Patience is key. For the time being, men can use proven treatments or adopt supportive measures (healthy routines, scalp care, etc.) while keeping an eye on reputable news about research developments.

Meanwhile, those who are happy with their current approach—whether it is medication, a hair transplant, or just a good haircut—may not need to jump at every new trend. If a truly transformative therapy emerges, doctors and media outlets will likely share that information widely.

Chapter 14: Important Nutrients and Dietary Factors

What you eat significantly affects how your body functions, including the health of your hair. While a balanced diet alone won't reverse genetic hair loss, poor nutrition can worsen shedding or breakage. Conversely, getting enough key vitamins, minerals, proteins, and fats can support stronger strands. For men aiming to keep as much hair as possible, or just wanting better-looking hair overall, focusing on food quality and nutrient intake is a wise move.

In this chapter, we will explore various dietary factors that affect hair and how to optimize them. We will also look at potential supplements and common deficiencies that may impact hair structure or the scalp environment. This information can guide you in making meal choices or deciding if you need extra help from vitamins or minerals.

14.1 The Role of Protein

14.1.1 Hair as a Protein Structure

Hair is mainly composed of a tough protein called keratin. Each strand grows from a hair follicle where new cells continually form and harden. If your diet lacks enough protein, the body may struggle to build healthy keratin. This can lead to weaker, thinner hair that is more prone to breakage.

14.1.2 Sources of Protein

- **Animal-Based:** Lean meats, poultry, fish, eggs, dairy. These offer complete protein with all essential amino acids.
- **Plant-Based:** Beans, lentils, tofu, tempeh, nuts, seeds. For those avoiding meat, combining different plant sources (e.g., rice and beans) can supply a full amino acid profile.

Men engaged in muscle-building often consume higher protein, which can also be beneficial for hair. However, extremely high protein diets paired with low overall nutrients might create imbalances. Moderation and variety are key.

14.2 Essential Vitamins and Their Impact

14.2.1 Vitamin A

Vitamin A helps the body produce sebum, an oily substance that keeps the scalp moisturized. A shortage of vitamin A can lead to a dry, itchy scalp. However, too much vitamin A has been linked to increased hair shedding, so it is important not to go overboard.

- **Sources:** Sweet potatoes, carrots, spinach, fish liver oil.
- **Signs of Excess:** Headaches, blurred vision, and hair loss if taken in very high amounts over time.

14.2.2 Vitamin C

Vitamin C supports the production of collagen, which helps maintain hair shaft strength. It also helps the body absorb iron (another key hair nutrient, discussed later). A shortage of vitamin C might lead to brittle hair.

- **Sources:** Citrus fruits (oranges, lemons), strawberries, bell peppers, broccoli.
- **Practical Tip:** Pair iron-rich foods with vitamin C foods to boost iron uptake.

14.2.3 Vitamin D

Research suggests a link between low vitamin D levels and certain types of hair thinning. Vitamin D might play a role in how follicles cycle through growth and rest stages.

- **Sources:** Sunlight exposure helps the skin make vitamin D. Also found in fatty fish, egg yolks, and fortified foods.

- **Supplement Caution:** Large doses can cause problems, so it's wise to check levels with a blood test before supplementing heavily.

14.2.4 Vitamin E

Vitamin E is an antioxidant that can help protect cells, including those in the scalp, from oxidative stress. Some small studies hint that it may promote healthier hair growth by reducing damage to follicles.

- **Sources:** Sunflower seeds, almonds, spinach, avocados.
- **Balance:** Excessive supplementation of vitamin E can thin the blood, so care is needed.

14.2.5 B Vitamins (Including Biotin)

The B vitamin family (like B12, folate, and biotin) assists with cell metabolism. Biotin specifically is often linked to hair health. True biotin deficiency is rare but can cause thinning or brittleness. Some men take high-dose biotin supplements, though extreme levels may not help if you are not actually deficient.

- **Sources:** Whole grains, eggs, dairy, meats, seeds, and nuts.
- **Practical Note:** Some men notice improved hair texture with modest biotin intake, but rely on a balanced diet first before jumping to large doses.

14.3 Key Minerals for Hair

14.3.1 Iron

Iron helps transport oxygen throughout the body, including to the scalp. Low iron (anemia) can cause hair to fall out or become weaker. While anemia is more common in women, men can also be low in iron due to poor diet or certain digestive conditions.

- **Sources:** Red meat, poultry, beans, lentils, leafy greens, fortified cereals.

- **Absorption Tip:** Combining plant-based iron with vitamin C (like squeezing lemon juice on spinach) can improve how much iron your body takes in.

14.3.2 Zinc

Zinc assists in tissue repair and helps keep oil glands around follicles working well. A lack of zinc may lead to hair shedding or a dry scalp. However, excessive zinc can disrupt the balance of other minerals like copper, so be cautious with supplements.

- **Sources:** Oysters, beef, pumpkin seeds, chickpeas.
- **Practical Note:** Some men see improvement in dandruff or scalp itching when correcting a mild zinc deficiency.

14.3.3 Selenium

Selenium supports various metabolic processes, including those affecting scalp health. Both deficiency and oversupply of selenium can cause brittle hair or changes in nails. It's best to stick to moderate amounts.

- **Sources:** Brazil nuts, seafood, whole grains.
- **Safety:** Just a few Brazil nuts can meet your daily selenium needs. Be mindful not to overeat them daily.

14.3.4 Magnesium

Magnesium is linked to hundreds of reactions in the body, some of which involve protein synthesis and hair growth. A shortage might indirectly slow hair-building processes, though severe deficiency is less common in well-balanced diets.

- **Sources:** Nuts, seeds, dark chocolate, whole grains.
- **Everyday Tip:** If stress is high, magnesium can also aid relaxation, which might indirectly support healthy hair by reducing stress-related shedding.

14.4 Healthy Fats and Hair Quality

1. **Omega-3 Fatty Acids:** Found in fatty fish (salmon, mackerel), walnuts, flaxseeds. These can reduce scalp dryness and inflammation.
2. **Omega-6 Fatty Acids:** Present in foods like sunflower oil or sesame seeds. Important too, but the typical Western diet often has too many omega-6 fats compared to omega-3.
3. **Monounsaturated Fats:** Avocados, olive oil, nuts. These can support overall health and help in keeping the scalp's oil balance stable.

Having a balanced ratio of these fats may create a better environment for hair growth. Extreme low-fat diets might lead to a lack of essential fatty acids, causing dryness or brittle strands.

14.5 Hydration and Its Importance

Hair can become more prone to breakage if the body is regularly dehydrated. While hair cells are not directly "hydrated" like skin, being low on fluid can reduce the body's ability to transport nutrients. A dehydrated scalp might also produce less of the healthy oils that keep hair supple.

- **Water Intake:** Aim for around 6-8 cups of fluid a day, depending on climate and activity.
- **Foods with High Water Content:** Fruits like watermelon or cucumbers can help maintain hydration levels.

14.6 Balancing Calories and Avoiding Extreme Diets

14.6.1 Crash Diets

When men try rapid weight loss, the body might perceive it as stress. This can prompt a condition like telogen effluvium, causing more hair to enter the resting phase and shed. Consistent, gradual weight management is less likely to shock the system.

14.6.2 Nutritional Gaps

Cutting out entire food groups without proper planning (for example, strict veganism without proper alternatives, or extremely low-carb diets without enough vegetables) can leave your body short on key vitamins and minerals. If you adopt a special diet, consult a nutrition expert or do thorough research to ensure you get all the basics needed for hair health.

14.7 Specific Diet Types and Hair Considerations

14.7.1 Plant-Based Diets (Vegan or Vegetarian)

Plant-based diets can support healthy hair if carefully balanced. It is important to secure enough protein, iron, zinc, and B12, which are often richer in animal sources. Men can look to fortified cereals, beans, lentils, nuts, seeds, and possibly supplements to fill gaps.

14.7.2 Low-Carb Diets

Men on low-carb or keto diets rely on higher fat and protein intake. While this can be okay for hair, if not balanced well, some men experience nutrient shortfalls or become low in vitamins found in certain fruits or whole grains. Monitoring micronutrient levels is essential.

14.7.3 Mediterranean-Style Eating

This approach includes a balance of whole grains, fruits, vegetables, fish, and healthy fats like olive oil. It naturally provides many nutrients linked to hair and overall well-being. Some studies hint that this type of diet could help maintain better scalp health and reduce inflammation.

14.8 Supplements: When and Why

14.8.1 Multivitamins

A daily multivitamin can act like an insurance policy if your diet is inconsistent. But not all multivitamins are the same. Look for ones with moderate doses of vitamins and minerals, not huge mega-doses.

14.8.2 Biotin Supplements

Biotin is popular for hair, though evidence of its effectiveness is stronger when a deficiency is present. High doses (like 5,000–10,000 mcg) are common in hair-targeted products, but if you already have normal biotin levels, the benefit may be small. Some men do report thicker hair or stronger nails with moderate biotin intake.

14.8.3 Collagen Peptides

Some men use collagen powders or gummies, hoping to support hair structure. Collagen is broken down in the digestive system, so direct hair benefits may vary. However, many users claim improvements in hair texture and strength. If you try these, choose a reputable brand and watch how you respond over several months.

14.8.4 Iron or Zinc Supplements

These should be guided by blood tests. Taking iron if you are not deficient can be harmful, since iron overload stresses the body. Similarly, too much zinc can disrupt mineral balance. Always confirm a deficiency or borderline level before supplementing.

14.9 Signs of Possible Nutritional Deficiencies Affecting Hair

- **Brittle or Dry Hair:** Could indicate a lack of healthy fats, certain vitamins, or dehydration.

- **Excessive Shedding:** Might be low iron or protein if medical causes have been ruled out.
- **Slow Growth Rate:** Nutrient shortfalls can delay the hair growth cycle.
- **Flaky or Itchy Scalp:** Could be linked to low vitamin A, zinc, or essential fatty acids.

For serious or sudden changes, consider seeing a dermatologist or doctor who can test for deficiencies or other medical conditions.

14.10 Does Diet Influence DHT or Hormones?

Since male pattern baldness is tied to DHT, men sometimes wonder if certain diets affect hormone levels. While no diet can block DHT to the degree of prescription medication, a generally healthy lifestyle can help balance overall hormone production and reduce chronic inflammation, which might aid scalp health.

- **Sugar and Refined Carbs:** High intake might raise insulin and possibly shift hormone balances. Some research ties insulin resistance to faster hair thinning in certain cases.
- **Balanced Fats:** Consuming moderate healthy fats could keep hormone production stable, rather than spiking or plummeting.
- **Moderate Weight Control:** Extreme obesity can affect hormones, including testosterone levels, which might in turn impact hair.

Thus, while diet alone is not a "cure" for androgen-driven hair loss, it can help create a stable environment in the body so that medical treatments or lifestyle measures work more effectively.

14.11 Combining Diet with Other Measures

1. **Medical Treatments:** If you're on minoxidil or finasteride, supporting hair growth with balanced meals might maximize the final result.

2. **Scalp Care Routines:** Good nutrition can reduce dryness or oiliness, aiding any topical treatments.
3. **Stress Management:** Nutrient-rich diets can support overall health, making the body more resilient against stress-induced shedding.
4. **Exercise and Sleep:** These also help regulate hormones and promote better circulation to the scalp.

Creating a synergy of diet, medication (if applicable), and daily hair care can lead to the best outcome for men worried about thinning.

14.12 Be Careful of "Miracle" Supplements

The marketplace is full of products promising instant regrowth through herbal blends or exotic roots. While some herbal elements might be mildly helpful, if a supplement's claims sound too good to be true (like "Regrow all lost hair in 2 weeks!"), they likely are. Any real improvement from diet changes or supplements generally takes months, since hair grows slowly.

If a supplement includes unclear ingredient lists or lacks reputable manufacturing details, it is wise to approach with caution. Stick to known brands or consult a doctor or dietitian before spending on pricey items that might not help—or could even harm you if they contain unknown chemicals.

14.13 Practical Tips for Building a Hair-Friendly Diet

- **Increase Variety:** Include colorful fruits and vegetables, lean proteins, whole grains, and healthy fats.
- **Snack Smart:** Replace chips or sweets with nuts, seeds, or yogurt for extra protein and micronutrients.
- **Hydration Habit:** Keep a water bottle handy. Start each morning with a glass of water to set the tone for the day.
- **Meal Planning:** Plan balanced meals rather than skipping or grabbing fast food often.

- **Moderate Supplements:** If you suspect a deficiency, get tested or seek professional guidance before high-dose supplementation.

14.14 Case Studies in Diet Improvement

1. **Case A:** A man in his 20s, who ate mostly fast food and sodas, noticed early thinning. Blood tests showed low iron and borderline low vitamin D. With a shift to more meat, leafy greens, and daily short sun exposure (plus a mild D supplement), his hair shedding slowed over six months, and he felt more energetic.
2. **Case B:** Another man on a strict vegetarian diet realized he wasn't getting enough protein. He added beans, lentils, tofu, and B12 supplements. Within a few months, his hair quality improved, and breakage reduced.
3. **Case C:** A busy professional tried to fix hair thinning with fancy products but ignored a sugar-heavy diet. After cutting back on sugary snacks and adding more whole foods, he felt less scalp irritation. While it didn't regrow lost hair, it seemed to reduce daily shedding.

These examples suggest that while diet is not a complete solution to heavy genetic hair loss, it can positively influence hair health when managed properly.

14.15 Monitoring and Adjusting

If you decide to shift your diet for hair health, track changes over time. Since hair grows slowly, it can take a couple of growth cycles (3-6 months) to notice improvements. Keep note of:

- **Shedding Levels:** Are you losing fewer strands during washing or brushing?
- **Scalp Condition:** Is flaking or dryness better?
- **Overall Energy:** Do you feel more balanced or healthy?

If no improvement occurs, or if hair loss continues rapidly, it might be time to consult a healthcare provider for further testing or explore other treatments.

14.16 Can Specific Foods Reverse Baldness?

No single food completely reverses male pattern hair loss. That process is highly driven by genetics and hormones. However, certain foods might strengthen the existing hair or reduce shedding caused by additional factors. A robust, nutrient-rich diet also helps treatments like finasteride or minoxidil do their best work, because your scalp and follicles receive steady support.

14.17 Balancing Lifestyle Beyond Diet

As repeated in prior chapters, many aspects of lifestyle come into play:

- **Stress Management:** Chronic stress can disrupt hormone levels and slow hair cell growth.
- **Adequate Sleep:** Nighttime is when many regenerative processes happen, including hair repair.
- **Regular Medical Checkups:** Catching issues like thyroid imbalances, anemia, or other internal problems early can limit their impact on hair.

Diet is a powerful part of the puzzle, but rarely stands alone as the only factor in hair health.

Chapter 15: Emotional Impact and Ways to Cope

Hair loss can be more than a simple physical change. It can affect a man's self-image, confidence, and emotional health, especially if the thinning or receding happens quickly. While some men easily adjust, others struggle with negative thoughts or worries about how they look. These feelings are valid. Recognizing the emotional side of hair loss is an important part of handling the issue in a healthy way.

This chapter focuses on the psychological effects that can come with thinning hair. We will explore why some men have a harder time coping than others, ways to manage stress or sadness, and what resources or support systems might be available. The goal is to offer practical pointers on how to address the emotional effects and move forward with more balance and calm.

15.1 Understanding the Emotional Side

15.1.1 Hair and Identity

Hair often holds symbolic or personal meaning. For many, it is linked to how youthful or confident they feel. It can also be a factor in cultural or family traditions. When hair starts thinning, it may seem like a clear sign of aging or losing control.

The emotional weight is not the same for everyone. Some men shrug off hair loss without much worry, while others feel upset or even angry. Neither reaction is "wrong." Emotional responses often tie in with how a man sees himself and what he finds important in his personal appearance.

15.1.2 Common Feelings

- **Fear:** Worry about looking older or less attractive.
- **Frustration:** Annoyed that one cannot easily stop the process.

- **Sadness:** Grieving the loss of a full head of hair that was once taken for granted.
- **Embarrassment:** Feeling self-conscious in social settings.

These reactions can be mild or strong, and they can change over time. For instance, a man might feel anxious when he first spots thinning, then gradually accept it, or vice versa.

15.2 Signs That Hair Loss Is Affecting Emotional Well-Being

Men who experience hair loss might see shifts in their mood or behavior. Examples include:

1. **Avoiding Social Events:** Fear of being teased or feeling "on display."
2. **Spending Excess Time in Mirrors:** Checking the hairline repeatedly or constantly comparing old photos.
3. **Mood Swings or Irritability:** Feeling upset or "on edge" because of concerns about looks.
4. **Frequent Negative Thoughts:** Telling oneself, "I'm less attractive," or "People are judging me."

At its extreme, hair loss worries can lead to a drop in self-esteem, anxiety in group settings, or even signs of depression if the individual feels hopeless. Recognizing these signs is the first step toward finding healthy ways to cope.

15.3 Why the Emotional Reaction Varies

15.3.1 Personal Values

A person who strongly values physical appearance or has a job that focuses on looks (like modeling, public speaking, or acting) may react more intensely. By contrast, someone who places less emphasis on hair might only be slightly concerned.

15.3.2 Age and Life Stage

Hair loss at a younger age (teens or early twenties) can be a shock. Men in older age groups sometimes handle it more calmly if they view it as a normal part of getting older. Still, this is not a rule; even men in their 50s can feel distressed.

15.3.3 Cultural Influences

Some cultures prize thick hair in males, linking it to strength or virility. Others may not stress hair as much. The more hair is seen as a sign of status, the more emotional the response can be.

15.3.4 Family and Peer Reactions

If friends or relatives tease a man about thinning hair, he might feel hurt. On the other hand, supportive remarks can help him manage any negative emotions.

15.4 Healthy Ways to Cope

15.4.1 Talking About It

Discussing hair loss worries with trusted friends, relatives, or a mental health professional can be a relief. It helps men see that they are not alone in their concerns. Some may find it easier to talk to a counselor who can offer ways to handle stress or negative self-image.

15.4.2 Staying Informed

Learning about the causes of hair loss, possible treatments, and realistic outcomes can reduce anxiety. Sometimes, fear comes from not knowing what is happening. Reading reliable information or talking to a professional can clarify how serious the issue is and what can be done.

15.4.3 Reframing Thoughts

Cognitive re-framing involves catching negative thoughts—like "People will think less of me because of my thinning hair"—and challenging them. Often, the reality is that others do not focus on our flaws as much as we think. Practicing a calmer, more balanced view can lower stress.

15.4.4 Exploring Styling or Treatment Options

Taking action, even in small ways, can help men feel more in control. This might be a new haircut that suits a receding hairline or trying proven treatments if desired. Choosing an approach (or choosing to do nothing) can feel more empowering than ignoring the situation completely.

15.5 Emotional Support Techniques

15.5.1 Relaxation Methods

Activities like gentle exercises, breathing exercises, or short calm sessions can reduce overall anxiety. Lower stress might also help reduce stress-related hair shedding (like telogen effluvium), though that depends on the individual case.

15.5.2 Physical Exercise

Regular physical activity is linked to better mood and lower tension. A short daily walk, a moderate run, or simple home workouts can produce endorphins that lift one's spirits. Exercise can also improve self-esteem by keeping the body healthy and fit.

15.5.3 Therapy or Counseling

Some men try counseling if they find the emotional weight is affecting their daily life. A trained counselor can give coping tools, help shift negative beliefs, and offer a safe place to discuss deeper worries. Therapy may be brief or long term, depending on personal preference.

15.5.4 Online or Local Groups

Support groups (online forums or local meetups) let men share stories, give tips on dealing with thinning hair, and realize many are going through the same experience. Reading success stories of how others adapted or found solutions can be reassuring.

15.6 Changing the Self-View

15.6.1 Focusing on Strengths

Feeling upset about hair loss can overshadow other positive traits—like kindness, sense of humor, or achievements. Making a point of noting these strengths can shift attention away from the thinning hair.

15.6.2 Considering a New Look

Some men who lose a large amount of hair decide to adopt a very short cut, like a buzz or even a fully shaved head. Surprisingly, many report feeling more self-confident once they fully commit to a new style instead of trying to hide thinning patches. This is a personal choice, but it can be freeing for those who are ready.

15.6.3 Building Self-Acceptance

Accepting hair loss does not mean giving up on oneself. It can mean acknowledging that it is happening and adjusting self-image to include this change. Some men discover that once they accept the new reality, they stop worrying as much about others' opinions and put that energy toward other parts of life.

15.7 Linking Emotions to Action

When hair loss starts, some men find a good way to cope emotionally is by taking concrete steps:

1. **Visit a Specialist:** Determine if the thinning is genetic or caused by another factor (stress, nutrient shortage, etc.).
2. **Plan a Routine:** Decide on daily or weekly habits, such as scalp care, better eating, or mild treatments.
3. **Set Realistic Goals:** Whether it is hair regrowth or simply a new hairstyle, having a target can make the process feel purposeful.

Taking action, even if hair regrowth is not the main priority, can offer psychological relief by turning a passive problem into an active project.

15.8 Family and Social Interactions

15.8.1 Talking to Loved Ones

Openly mentioning concerns about hair loss can lessen misunderstandings. Close friends or partners can be supportive if they understand the level of worry. They might offer new perspectives, encourage professional help, or even help pick a new hairstyle.

15.8.2 Handling Teasing or Remarks

Casual teasing from friends can sometimes hurt more than intended. Some men find it useful to calmly express that such jokes bother them. Others respond with humor or simply let the comments pass if they do not sting. The best approach depends on personality and how serious the teasing is.

15.9 When Is Professional Help Needed?

Not every man dealing with thinning hair needs therapy. But if one notices:

- **Prolonged Sadness:** Feeling down for weeks without lifting.
- **Social Withdrawal:** Avoiding most or all social interactions.
- **Persistent Anxiety:** Ongoing nervousness or fear about appearance.
- **Disruption in Daily Life:** Trouble sleeping, eating, or focusing.

...it might be wise to see a counselor, psychologist, or doctor. Hair loss might not be the only factor—other life stresses could be involved. A professional can help untangle these problems.

15.10 Success Stories and Different Paths

It can help to see how other men have managed the emotional challenge of thinning hair:

1. **Case A:** A man in his late 20s noticed a receding hairline, felt panic, and started avoiding social outings. He spoke with a counselor who helped him see that most peers did not judge him by his hair. He later tried a short haircut, discovered he liked the look, and regained confidence.
2. **Case B:** Another man tried many treatments without much change, felt depressed, and eventually sought therapy. Realizing that his self-worth need not depend on hair, he chose to focus on fitness and good nutrition. He found he still cared about hair, but it was no longer the center of his self-image.
3. **Case C:** A man tried medical treatments early, saw partial improvement, and found this was enough to boost his optimism. He joined an online forum where he exchanged tips and felt supported. Over time, he accepted that mild thinning might continue, but felt good about doing what he could.

Each path is unique. Some men find relief in acceptance, others prefer to pursue treatments, and still others combine both approaches.

Chapter 16: Debunking Common Myths

In the realm of hair loss, myths are plentiful. From old legends about wearing hats to modern claims of miracle cures, confusion can arise. These myths can lead men astray, prompt the use of ineffective or harmful products, or create unnecessary worry. Understanding the facts is a big step in making smart choices about hair care and hair loss treatments.

This chapter exposes several popular myths and provides accurate information to replace them. By separating truth from fiction, men can avoid wasting time and money, or worsening an issue that might be better managed through proven methods.

16.1 Myth 1: Wearing Hats Causes Baldness

A very common belief is that frequent hat use leads to thinning hair. The idea often goes that the scalp "cannot breathe" or that the constant friction of a hat pulls hair out.

16.1.1 Reality

- **Oxygen and Follicles:** Hair follicles get their oxygen from blood, not air around them. Wearing a hat does not cut off oxygen to the follicles.
- **Friction:** If a hat is extremely tight, it could irritate the scalp, but typical hats do not apply enough tension to damage follicles.
- **Hygiene:** A dirty hat might lead to scalp issues or infections if rarely washed, which can cause some local irritation, but not true pattern baldness.

In short, normal hat-wearing does not cause permanent hair loss. However, if a man notices scalp irritation, switching to a looser or cleaner hat can help.

16.2 Myth 2: Only Older Men Lose Their Hair

People sometimes assume baldness is only a problem for men in their 40s, 50s, or beyond.

16.2.1 Reality

- **Early Onset:** Some men notice a receding hairline in late teens or early twenties.
- **Genetic Factors:** Certain genetic patterns can trigger male pattern baldness at younger ages.
- **Life Events:** Stress, poor diet, or medical conditions can cause shedding at any point in adulthood.

Hair loss can indeed happen in older men, but it does not wait for a specific age. Young men can also face thinning, which can be emotionally challenging if they are not prepared for it.

16.3 Myth 3: Cutting Hair Frequently Makes It Grow Thicker

This myth arises from the idea that hair appears thicker after a fresh trim. Many believe that shaving or cutting hair more often will encourage stronger or faster growth.

16.3.1 Reality

- **Hair Structure:** Cutting hair changes only the shaft above the scalp, not the growth process below the scalp.
- **Visual Effect:** Newly cut hair can appear thicker or less wispy, but the actual diameter of each strand or the rate of growth does not change.
- **Regular Trims:** While beneficial for reducing split ends and making hair look healthier, they do not alter follicle function.

If thinning is caused by genetics or hormones, no amount of trimming will slow or reverse it. Trims do help hair look tidier, but they do not fix the root issue.

16.4 Myth 4: Stress Is the Main Reason for Hair Loss

There is a common assumption that anyone losing hair must be under too much stress.

16.4.1 Reality

- **Androgenetic Alopecia:** The most frequent cause is genetic, tied to hormones like DHT, not simply stress.
- **Stress-Linked Shedding:** Telogen effluvium can happen after major events (illness, surgery, or emotional trauma), but it usually causes temporary shedding, not long-term pattern hair loss.
- **Multiple Causes:** Nutritional deficits, immune system issues, or harsh styling can also contribute. Stress is just one factor among many.

Reducing stress is good for general health and might help if hair is in a reactive shedding phase, but it cannot singlehandedly resolve genetic hair thinning.

16.5 Myth 5: Daily Hair Washing Leads to Greater Shedding

Some believe that each wash causes hair to fall out, so they reduce shampooing to prevent loss.

16.5.1 Reality

- **Visible Strands in the Shower:** It might look like more hair is falling out, but these are typically strands already in the shedding

phase. If they did not fall in the shower, they would appear on a pillow or comb.
- **Healthy Scalp:** Regular but gentle washing keeps the scalp clean, which might even help in cases of excess oil or dandruff.
- **Over-Washing Caution:** Using very harsh shampoos too frequently can irritate the scalp, but it does not usually cause permanent hair loss—just breakage or dryness.

Men can adjust washing frequency based on scalp type (oily, normal, dry), but moderate washing with a mild shampoo is fine.

16.6 Myth 6: Using Gel or Styling Products Causes Baldness

Another myth is that hair gel or wax seeps into follicles and kills them.

16.6.1 Reality

- **Surface-Level Application:** Styling products stay mostly on the hair shaft, not inside the follicle.
- **Scalp Buildup:** Leaving heavy products unwashed for long periods can clog pores, possibly causing irritation. However, this is not the same as genetic hair loss.
- **Patchy Issues:** If a scalp reacts badly to certain chemicals, it might cause redness or mild hair shedding. In general, though, normal use of common styling items does not produce long-term thinning.

It is wise to rinse out heavy products before bed to keep the scalp healthy, but men do not need to give up gels or waxes out of baldness worries.

16.7 Myth 7: Supplements Guarantee Regrowth

Countless supplements claim to "reverse balding" or "grow hair fast." People often assume a pill can solve everything.

16.7.1 Reality

- **Nutrient Deficiencies:** Hair can suffer if a man lacks protein, vitamins, or minerals. Correcting a shortage can help. However, most men with a balanced diet are not severely lacking.
- **Genetic Loss Remains:** Supplements may improve overall hair condition but rarely fix the underlying genetic pattern.
- **Beware "Miracle" Claims:** Aggressive marketing often misleads. Real results take months, and no pill can fully defeat genetic hair loss.

Supplements can be helpful if there is a proven deficiency or a borderline case. Otherwise, they should be seen as supportive, not a magic fix.

16.8 Myth 8: Massage Alone Can Stop Baldness

Scalp massage feels pleasant and may boost blood flow. Some say it alone can halt male pattern hair loss.

16.8.1 Reality

- **Circulation:** While massage may increase blood flow, the underlying hormonal sensitivity of follicles remains if it is genetic.
- **Stress Relief:** Massage can reduce tension, which might lower stress-related shedding. But for androgenetic alopecia, it does not solve the DHT issue.
- **Combination Approach:** Including scalp massage in a broader routine (using mild oils, for instance) may support scalp health, but expecting it to end genetic loss is unrealistic.

Enjoying massage is fine, yet it should not be counted on as the sole method to combat pattern baldness.

16.9 Myth 9: Plucking Gray Hairs Results in More Gray or Thin Hairs

People often say if you pluck one gray hair, two or three will appear in its place.

16.9.1 Reality

- **Hair Color and Growth Cycle:** Plucking a gray hair just removes that one strand. It does not change neighboring follicles.
- **Possible Follicle Damage:** Repeated plucking can damage the follicle, possibly leading to less or no hair growth in that spot over time.
- **Genetics of Graying:** Hair color is genetically controlled; plucking does not alter this progression.

So, plucking gray hairs will not trigger new patches of gray or cause widespread thinning, though it can irritate the scalp if done repeatedly.

16.10 Myth 10: Only Mothers Pass on Baldness Genes

It is often repeated that a man inherits baldness solely from his maternal grandfather's side.

16.10.1 Reality

- **Polygenic Trait:** Hair loss can come from both sides of the family, involving multiple genes.
- **Father's Influence:** Some men mirror their father's pattern more than their mother's side, or a mix.
- **Predicting is Hard:** Even if one side has no hair loss, genes from several generations back can still appear.

While a strong maternal link might exist in some lines, it is not an exclusive rule. Looking at both sides of the family (and extended relatives) gives a fuller picture.

16.11 Myth 11: Sunlight Directly Causes Hair to Fall

Some believe that exposing the scalp to too much sun kills follicles.

16.11.1 Reality

- **UV Damage:** Excess sun can burn the scalp, leading to dryness or short-term breakage. It does not directly cause typical male pattern thinning.
- **Care in Harsh Sun:** Using a light sunscreen or wearing a hat can protect against burns, which are more noticeable if hair is thin.
- **Long-Term Risk:** Chronic sun damage could weaken the skin over time, but does not usually trigger complete bald spots unless severe.

Men should protect the scalp from sunburn for comfort and skin health, but normal sun exposure is not a direct cause of hair loss.

16.12 Myth 12: Medications Make Hair Loss Worse Before It Gets Better

Some confusion surrounds the "shedding phase" linked with treatments like minoxidil, leading to rumors that these medicines worsen baldness.

16.12.1 Reality

- **Shedding Phase Explained:** When starting certain treatments, some older hairs in the resting phase may fall out early, clearing the way for stronger, new growth.
- **Temporary Effect:** This initial shed usually stops within weeks, then hair growth can pick up.
- **Long-Term Benefit:** If consistent usage is maintained, many see thicker coverage or at least slower loss.

Thinking that meds cause permanent harm is not correct. Sticking with a treatment plan can yield positive results for many men.

16.13 Myth 13: Hair Loss Has No Effect on Health

Some assume that hair loss is just a cosmetic matter and never signals an underlying problem.

16.13.1 Reality

- **Possible Signals:** Sometimes, shedding can reflect thyroid issues, low iron, autoimmune disorders, or high stress.
- **Health Checks:** If sudden or patchy shedding occurs, a medical evaluation might uncover a correctable factor.
- **Mental Health:** Chronic worry about hair loss can affect emotional well-being, as noted in the previous chapter.

While standard male pattern loss is often harmless physically, ignoring potential medical or emotional factors could be unwise.

16.14 Myth 14: Hair Transplants Produce Immediate Results

Some men think a transplant fixes the problem right away, walking out of the clinic with a full head of hair the next day.

16.14.1 Reality

- **Procedure and Healing:** After surgery, scabs form, and the transplanted hairs often shed within a few weeks. Then, new growth can take several months.
- **Final Look:** Results usually become clear at 6-12 months post-operation.
- **Maintenance:** Men might still need medication to protect non-transplanted follicles from future thinning.

Expecting instant fullness leads to disappointment. Patience is essential when dealing with transplants.

16.15 Myth 15: Every Hair Loss Treatment Is a Scam

Skepticism is healthy, but some people swing to the other extreme and assume nothing works.

16.15.1 Reality

- **Proven Treatments:** Finasteride, minoxidil, and certain transplant methods do have positive track records for many men.
- **Variability:** Results vary. Some get great outcomes, others see moderate improvement, and a few do not respond well.
- **Scams Do Exist:** There are indeed fake cures and questionable products, so research is key.

The presence of scams does not mean all treatments are useless. Finding recognized methods and consulting a professional can lead to real benefits.

16.16 Myth 16: Brushing the Scalp 100 Times a Day Prevents Hair Loss

An older idea suggests that constant brushing stimulates follicles enough to keep hair from falling out.

16.16.1 Reality

- **Breakage Risk:** Over-brushing can stress and break hair.
- **Blood Flow:** Light brushing might boost circulation, but not enough to counteract hormonal hair loss.
- **Scalp Condition:** Gently removing tangles is good, but excessive brushing can irritate the scalp.

A normal brushing routine is enough. Telling people to brush hair 100 times daily is outdated and can cause damage if done harshly.

16.17 Spotting Reliable Information

To avoid falling for myths:

- **Check Reputable Sources:** Look for scientific journals, dermatologist websites, or well-known medical clinics.
- **Consult Specialists:** A hair loss expert or dermatologist can explain the cause of a man's thinning and propose sensible options.
- **Ask Questions:** If a claim seems extreme—like guaranteeing a full head of hair in a week—be cautious.
- **Avoid Panic:** Myths can spark anxiety. Stay calm, gather facts, and decide on next steps with a level head.

16.18 Leveraging Accurate Knowledge

By dispelling myths, men can:

1. **Focus on Real Solutions:** Instead of trying worthless products or methods.
2. **Save Money and Time:** Avoiding scams or unproven schemes.
3. **Reduce Worry:** Understanding that many common tales of hair loss are exaggerated or wrong.
4. **Take Action Wisely:** Considering established treatments, adopting a balanced lifestyle, or deciding to accept hair changes.

Learning the facts helps men make better choices for their well-being, both physically and emotionally.

Chapter 17: Building a Support Network

Hair loss can feel like a private matter, but the reality is that many men face the same challenge. Reaching out to others and sharing experiences can make a big difference. A solid support system—whether it involves friends, family, professionals, or online groups—can be the key to handling the emotional and practical aspects of thinning hair.

In this chapter, we will discuss the value of a strong support network for men dealing with hair loss. We will look at different types of support, ways to find reliable connections, and tips on forming and maintaining helpful relationships. The goal is to guide readers on how to lean on others in a healthy way, ask for assistance when needed, and return the favor by helping others in the same boat.

17.1 Why Support Matters

17.1.1 Shared Understanding

Hair loss can bring up concerns about appearance, self-worth, and identity. Talking with people who have gone through similar feelings can ease worries. When someone else confirms, "I felt the same way," it can reduce the sense of isolation.

17.1.2 Emotional Relief

A good support network allows men to express frustration or sadness in a safe space. Simply voicing these emotions can reduce anxiety and build confidence. By comparing notes, men learn that hair loss does not have to ruin quality of life or personal image.

17.1.3 Practical Tips

Networking with others often brings out real-life tricks that might not appear in textbooks: how to style thinning hair, how to talk to a barber, which clinics are trustworthy, and which products or routines might work for a particular hair type. Firsthand advice can help men avoid trial-and-error approaches.

17.2 Types of Support Networks

17.2.1 Family and Close Friends

The simplest form of support often comes from the people we see every day. They may already care deeply about your well-being. However, not everyone feels comfortable discussing hair loss with family, especially if relatives have strong opinions or might tease. If family or close friends are understanding, they can be a big help—giving honest feedback about new haircuts or simply listening to concerns.

17.2.2 Professional Counselors or Therapists

For some, hair loss can trigger substantial stress, anxiety, or low mood. Meeting with a counselor or therapist provides a setting to explore these emotions in depth. A mental health professional can offer coping strategies, help reduce negative self-talk, and possibly identify other areas of life that are fueling stress-related hair shedding. Even a handful of sessions can be revealing.

17.2.3 Local Support Groups

Cities may have face-to-face meetups or groups focused on hair loss. This can be arranged by hair clinics, community centers, or general men's health initiatives. Attending a local group lets participants talk in person, share stories, compare product experiences, and see that the issue is very common. A sense of belonging often develops.

17.2.4 Online Forums and Communities

In the digital era, many men turn to internet boards or social media groups dedicated to hair loss topics. These platforms are convenient for those in remote areas or who prefer some privacy. Participants can read threads, ask questions, and browse before-and-after pictures. However, not all online spaces are created equal. Checking the credibility of the advice is essential, as misinformation can be common.

17.2.5 Medical Professionals

Dermatologists, trichologists, and hair restoration specialists can be part of a broader support network. Beyond diagnosing causes and recommending treatments, they can offer encouragement, monitor progress, and adapt plans as needed. A trusting relationship with a specialist can remove some of the uncertainty tied to hair loss.

17.3 Finding the Right Environment

17.3.1 Comfort and Openness

A support network works only if members feel safe and accepted. Whether the group is face-to-face or online, it is crucial that discussions remain respectful. If a particular forum is full of insults or negativity, it may do more harm than good. Spending time in places that encourage open conversation and understanding is key.

17.3.2 Shared Interests or Demographics

Some men seek groups tailored to their age range or background. For instance, a younger man might want a group of peers who began losing hair in their twenties, while an older man might connect with those who have a different perspective. Groups can also focus on different aspects: some are purely about product and treatment tips, while others focus on emotional well-being or acceptance.

17.3.3 Checking Reliability

With online communities, it is easy for anyone to post untested claims. Before following advice about supplements, medications, or unusual remedies, look for scientific backing or consult a medical professional. A community's success stories can be inspiring, but be sure to separate personal anecdotes from proven facts.

17.4 How to Engage in a Supportive Way

17.4.1 Sharing Your Story

When first joining a group—online or in person—introduce yourself. Mention your type of hair loss (if known), how long you have dealt with it, and what your goals are. Being open can encourage others to do the same, sparking helpful discussions.

17.4.2 Asking Direct Questions

If you need feedback on a particular product, routine, or clinic, pose direct questions. This way, the group can respond in a focused manner. For example: "Has anyone used Product X for hair thickening? How long did it take to see results?" can yield more targeted replies than a vague "Any tips on hair thickening?"

17.4.3 Giving Feedback

Supporting others is part of building a strong network. If you have tried a method that worked (or did not work), share your honest experiences. Keep the tone respectful and constructive, especially if your viewpoint differs from someone else's. Avoid belittling remarks or personal attacks.

17.4.4 Respecting Boundaries

People have different comfort levels in discussing personal topics. Some might be eager to post photos of their hairline changes; others may prefer to keep that private. Do not pressure anyone to reveal details they are not ready to share.

17.5 Benefits of One-on-One Connections

17.5.1 Accountability Buddies

Rather than relying solely on large communities, forming a one-on-one bond can help sustain motivation. For instance, if two men are both trying a new medication or scalp routine, they might update each other weekly, compare notes, and ensure consistency.

17.5.2 Emotional Check-Ins

A close friend or fellow forum member can become a go-to person for emotional check-ins. Sharing small wins (like noticing less shedding) or frustrations (such as a new patch of thinning) can be easier in a private message than a public group.

17.5.3 Trust and Honesty

Over time, one-on-one relationships can build deeper trust, enabling more candid discussions. It is also easier to share personal updates about mental health or how hair loss might be affecting relationships or work, without worrying about judgement from strangers.

17.6 Family Support: Navigating Complex Reactions

17.6.1 Different Family Perspectives

In families with multiple generations of hair loss, relatives may have strong opinions. A father who managed baldness at a young age might brush off concerns with, "It's no big deal, just accept it," while a mother might be more worried about her son's emotional state. Understanding these varied perspectives can help reduce family conflicts.

17.6.2 Setting Boundaries

If teasing from siblings or relatives becomes hurtful, it might help to state clearly: "I'd prefer if you didn't joke about my hair. It makes me uncomfortable." People who care about you will hopefully respect that boundary once it is voiced.

17.6.3 Letting Loved Ones Help

Sometimes men feel they must handle hair loss alone. But involving supportive family members can ease the journey. A sibling might recommend a reputable clinic, or a partner might help apply scalp treatments or remind you of medication times. Collaboration can lighten the emotional load.

17.7 Building Confidence Through Shared Activities

17.7.1 Group Initiatives

Support networks can extend beyond discussions. Some local groups organize activities—like attending a men's health fair, going to a hair-loss-related expo, or trying out group fitness classes. Engaging in these events can build camaraderie and demonstrate that hair loss does not limit life experiences.

17.7.2 Workshops and Seminars

Medical centers or health clubs sometimes hold workshops on scalp care, stress management, or nutrition for better hair. Attending these with a friend or group allows for learning in a supportive environment. Plus, group members can compare what they learned afterward to decide which tips are most practical.

17.8 Technology and Online Support Platforms

17.8.1 Video Meetups

Online video tools let people connect from different regions. Virtual meetings can bring face-to-face interactions without the need to travel.

Some men find it more personal than text-only forums, though it requires stable internet and willingness to appear on camera.

17.8.2 Anonymous Chat Apps

For those who are shy or want to keep hair loss private, anonymous apps or forums can provide a safe space. Users can choose a nickname and share experiences without revealing their true identity. This can be a starting point before deciding if one wants to meet others in person.

17.8.3 Dedicated Hair Loss Platforms

Aside from general social media, some platforms are specialized for hair loss discussions. They might offer features like progress-tracking photo galleries, private messaging, product reviews, and a Q&A section with verified professionals. This can streamline the search for information.

17.9 Staying Grounded

17.9.1 Balancing Advice With Personal Judgment

A broad support network means many opinions. What works for one person might fail for another. While listening to success stories is helpful, each man's situation is unique. Combine peer advice with professional input to avoid chasing unproven methods or quick fixes.

17.9.2 Handling Negative Comments

Unfortunately, any public forum can attract negativity or trolling. If someone criticizes or mocks, remember that their words do not define you. Use blocking or reporting features if needed. A well-moderated group usually has rules to prevent disrespectful behavior.

17.10 Overcoming Barriers to Seeking Support

17.10.1 Pride or Embarrassment

Some men feel that asking for help or discussing hair loss is a sign of weakness. Overcoming this mindset is the first step to relief. Hair loss is a common, natural occurrence, and reaching out is a normal way to cope with challenges.

17.10.2 Fear of Judgment

Worry that others will make fun can be a stumbling block. However, in supportive environments, many men realize that others are kind and eager to help. The fear of judgment is often larger in the mind than in reality.

17.10.3 Time Constraints

Busy schedules can hinder joining groups or reading forums. If time is tight, even a brief check-in once a week can maintain a sense of community. Some men schedule a regular message with a friend or set aside 10 minutes daily to browse a helpful forum.

17.11 Case Examples

1. **Case A:** Mark, age 35, began losing hair around the crown. He felt alone, so he joined a local men's health club that met monthly. Through new connections, he learned about scalp micropigmentation and felt more comfortable exploring it, because he trusted firsthand accounts from others in the group.
2. **Case B:** James, age 25, turned to an online forum. Initially, he only read posts. After seeing many supportive responses, he posted a photo of his hairline and got honest, friendly feedback about styling and possible treatments. Encouraged, James also found an accountability buddy for minoxidil usage, which boosted his commitment.

3. **Case C:** Robert, in his 40s, was anxious about family teasing. He spoke to a counselor who guided him on how to set boundaries with well-meaning but overly blunt relatives. He also learned stress-reduction techniques, noticing an improvement in his overall mood.

17.12 Giving Back to the Community

Support networks work best when members both receive and offer help. After you gain knowledge or confidence, you may find that you can encourage newcomers. This reciprocity reinforces the positive atmosphere. Sharing your successes (and your failures) can prevent others from making the same missteps.

Chapter 18: Tools and Technology for Hair Loss

Modern times have seen significant progress in technology geared toward hair care and hair loss monitoring. From specialized devices used by dermatologists to phone apps for at-home tracking, there is a growing range of tools that men can use to gain insights into their scalp health and manage thinning hair more effectively.

In this chapter, we will examine some of the common and emerging technologies in hair loss support. We will break down how these tools work, their potential benefits, and any drawbacks or limitations they may have. Whether someone wants to keep track of their hairline over months or delve into advanced therapies, understanding these technologies can make it easier to choose the right solutions.

18.1 Home Monitoring and Tracking Apps

18.1.1 Photography-Based Apps

One simple yet effective approach is using apps that help users take consistent, well-lit photos of their hair over time. By positioning the camera at the same angle and lighting conditions, men can visually track changes month by month. These apps may feature:

- **Guided Outlines:** Onscreen guides show where to align the scalp for comparison shots.
- **Side-by-Side Galleries:** Users can view pictures from different points in time to spot subtle shifts.
- **Reminders:** Notifications to take photos at set intervals.

While such apps do not actively treat hair loss, they give a clearer sense of whether existing routines or medications are working. People often over- or underestimate changes when relying on memory alone.

18.1.2 Hair Loss Logs and Calendars

Some apps function like diaries, letting users record details: day's hair shedding level, stress factors, diet notes, or medication usage. Patterns may emerge, revealing triggers or improvements. For instance, if a user sees more shedding after a week of poor sleep or missed medication doses, they can adjust habits accordingly.

18.1.3 Caution With Self-Diagnosis

Though apps can be handy, relying solely on digital self-assessment has limits. If the app suggests a certain condition without professional input, it could cause unnecessary worry or lead to ignoring a more serious problem. Using these platforms along with medical advice is recommended.

18.2 Handheld Scalp Analyzers

18.2.1 What Are They?

These are devices, often resembling small wands or cameras, that magnify and capture images of scalp and hair follicles. They can reveal details not visible to the naked eye—like miniaturized hairs, clogged pores, or the presence of dryness or oiliness.

18.2.2 Who Uses Them?

- **Clinics:** Professionals use high-end versions to examine patterns of thinning, measure follicle diameter, or diagnose scalp conditions.
- **Consumers:** Some companies sell affordable home models, though the quality may be lower than clinical-grade. They can still offer a closer look than a simple mirror.

18.2.3 Possible Benefits

- **Early Detection:** Pinpoint areas of thinning at a stage when the issue is less visible.

- **Monitoring Progress:** Compare images before and after treatments.
- **Scalp Health Check:** Spot potential issues (like dandruff or mild infections) early on.

18.2.4 Limitations

- **Learning Curve:** Interpreting magnified images requires some knowledge. Users might misread normal variations as problems.
- **Cost Variations:** High-quality devices can be pricey, while cheaper ones might be less accurate.

18.3 Laser and Light-Based Devices

18.3.1 Low-Level Laser Therapy (LLLT)

Already discussed briefly in earlier chapters, LLLT devices—such as laser combs, caps, or helmets—emit light energy that may stimulate blood flow and cellular activity in hair follicles. Many men use them at home, wearing a laser cap for a few sessions each week.

- **Convenience:** Some caps allow hands-free use while doing other tasks.
- **Consistent Use Needed:** Stopping can lead to a return to prior shedding levels.
- **Varying Results:** Some see positive outcomes, while others notice little change.

18.3.2 Light-Emitting Diodes (LED)

LED therapy is similar to LLLT but uses different wavelengths and lower intensities. Some scalp treatment centers offer LED sessions, aiming to reduce inflammation and possibly promote mild regrowth. The at-home market is smaller for pure LED hair devices compared to laser caps.

18.3.3 Precautions

While many find these devices harmless, overuse or incorrect usage could cause scalp irritation or headaches. Always follow manufacturer guidelines and, if unsure, ask a specialist for advice.

18.4 Scalp Micropigmentation (SMP) Equipment

18.4.1 The Process

SMP involves using special tattoo machines that deposit tiny dots of pigment on the scalp, creating the illusion of hair stubble or added density among existing strands. It is a non-surgical cosmetic procedure that requires skill to look natural.

18.4.2 Technological Aspects

Modern SMP machines allow precise control over needle depth and pigment flow, which reduces pain and speeds healing. Some clinics also use computerized systems that map the scalp to ensure even pigment distribution.

18.4.3 Points to Consider

- **Maintenance:** Pigment can fade over years, needing touch-ups.
- **Realistic Results:** If done well, it can look quite convincing at a short distance, but not like long, flowing hair.
- **Operator Expertise:** Technology matters, but the artist's skill is equally critical. Inexperienced hands can produce blotchy results.

18.5 Advanced Clinical Tools

18.5.1 Platelet-Rich Plasma (PRP) Kits

Clinics use specialized centrifuges to create PRP from a patient's blood. This concentrated platelet mix is then injected into thinning areas. The process relies on precise equipment to separate platelet layers effectively. While results vary, many see improvements in thickness or reduced shedding over multiple sessions.

18.5.2 Robotic Hair Transplant Systems

Some hair transplant centers use robotic devices to assist with follicle extraction and graft placement. These systems can pinpoint and harvest grafts with precision, potentially reducing human error. They also:

- **Analyze Donor Areas:** Evaluate follicle angles and choose the best grafts.
- **Minimize Scarring:** By using small punches more consistently than manual approaches.
- **Streamline Procedures:** Surgeons oversee the robot, but the technology handles mechanical repetition.

However, robots are tools, not replacements for a skilled surgeon. Experience still guides planning, hairline design, and finishing touches.

18.6 Virtual Consultations and Telehealth

18.6.1 Remote Assessments

Some clinics offer video consultations for hair loss. The patient shares photos or uses a live camera to show their scalp. A specialist can then provide an initial opinion, suggest blood tests, or recommend a treatment plan. This helps men who live far from specialized centers or prefer not to travel.

18.6.2 App-Based Prescriptions

In certain regions, health apps partner with licensed doctors who prescribe medications like finasteride or minoxidil after an online exam. The medication is then shipped directly. This convenience appeals to those who find in-person visits time-consuming or stressful.

18.6.3 Responsible Use

Remote services are handy, but they may miss details that an in-person exam would catch. A telehealth doctor might not spot scalp conditions or subtle signs. If the hair loss is complex or unusual, an in-person follow-up may be necessary.

18.7 Personalized Data Tracking

18.7.1 Wearable Tech?

While not yet mainstream, there is talk of wearable devices that could measure scalp temperature or sweat composition to glean insights about stress or local inflammation. This could, in theory, correlate with shedding patterns. However, practical consumer versions remain limited.

18.7.2 Smart Combs or Brushes

Some companies have experimented with "smart brushes" that track brushing habits, measure hair dryness, or detect breakage. The device usually syncs with a phone app for suggestions (like adjusting styling frequency or using conditioner more often). While innovative, many users find these novelty-like or too costly for the benefits offered.

18.8 Assessing the Cost and Benefit

18.8.1 Budget Considerations

Home devices like laser caps can cost several hundred to over a thousand dollars. Robotic transplants can be pricier than manual methods. Even scalp analyzers vary widely in price. Before investing, weigh how central the device or procedure is to your goals. Could the money be better spent on proven medications or consultations?

18.8.2 Evidence of Effectiveness

Always look for real clinical studies or credible reviews. Some brands do extensive research; others rely on marketing hype. Checking professional forums, dermatologist recommendations, or trusted health websites can clarify whether a product is backed by solid data.

18.9 Safety Measures and Maintenance

18.9.1 Device Upkeep

For physical equipment (like scalp analyzers or laser helmets), follow cleaning and storage instructions. Dirty or damaged devices can lead to incorrect readings, scalp irritation, or less effective sessions.

18.9.2 Following Instructions Strictly

Misusing a device—such as applying laser therapy too long or skipping recommended intervals—may lead to side effects or no benefit. Overuse sometimes irritates the skin, while underuse will not yield results. Consistency is key with technology-based treatments.

18.10 Combining Technology With Conventional Treatments

18.10.1 Monitoring Medication Progress

Apps and scalp analyzers can track how well finasteride, minoxidil, or other meds are working. By comparing photos or measurement data over months, men can see if a new routine actually delivers results.

18.10.2 Laser Therapy and Topicals

Some men use laser devices along with minoxidil or other topical agents. The laser might improve circulation, helping the scalp absorb the medication more thoroughly. However, confirm with a doctor that it is safe to combine them.

18.11 Case Examples of Tech Use

1. **Case A:** Chris invests in a laser cap after reading decent reviews. He uses it for 20 minutes, three times a week, while continuing oral finasteride. He also takes monthly scalp photos with a dedicated app. Over six months, images show moderate thickening around the crown, reinforcing that his combined approach is working.
2. **Case B:** Samuel tries a cheaper handheld scalp analyzer to monitor dryness and see if his new anti-dandruff shampoo helps. With magnified images, he spots reduced flaking after a few weeks. He shares these images on an online forum for feedback from others who have tried the same shampoo.
3. **Case C:** Trevor undergoes a robotic FUE transplant. The clinic's system maps his donor area, extracting grafts with uniform precision. After the surgery, he uses an app to remind him of post-op care steps, track healing, and upload photos for the surgeon to review virtually. This synergy of technology helps him feel informed at every stage.

18.12 Pitfalls and Warnings

- **Misleading Ads:** Some products display exaggerated testimonials or doctored photos. Be skeptical.
- **Overdependence on Devices:** Technology can help track progress but does not automatically solve root causes.
- **Lack of Clinical Validation:** Many consumer gadgets skip rigorous testing, so their claims may be anecdotal.
- **Privacy Concerns:** Apps that store photos or personal data could pose privacy risks if not properly encrypted.

18.13 The Future of Hair Tech

Beyond what is currently available, researchers are exploring:

- **AI-Driven Diagnostics:** Apps that use machine learning to compare your scalp images with huge databases, offering more precise suggestions.
- **3D Scalp Printing:** Some labs dream of "printing" new follicle structures that could be transplanted. This is still in experimental stages.
- **Gene Therapy Delivery Systems:** Micro-robots or nano-carriers that deliver gene-editing tools right to the follicles, though this remains highly theoretical.

While these sound promising, they may take years to become a reality. Men should focus on what is proven or at least has credible data behind it if they want results now.

18.14 Tips for Selecting Technology

1. **Consult Pros:** Before buying expensive laser caps or scalp analyzers, ask a dermatologist if such devices fit your hair loss type.
2. **Test Return Policies:** If allowed, try the product for a set time. Some companies give partial refunds if no improvement is seen.
3. **Avoid Overly Flashy Claims:** "Guaranteed to regrow lost hair in 2 weeks!" is likely false. Real solutions need patience.
4. **Seek Real Reviews:** Check multiple sources, including verified purchase reviews or medical community feedback.

18.15 Integrating Technology Into a Daily or Weekly Routine

- **Set Reminders:** Use phone alarms to schedule laser therapy sessions or scalp check pictures.

- **Track Consistently:** Weekly or monthly intervals often strike a good balance between detail and convenience.
- **Share With Specialists:** If you have a dermatologist, bring your app data or device images to appointments. It helps them see how your condition evolves.

18.16 Balancing Tech With Lifestyle

Tools and tech alone cannot beat genetic hair loss if broader lifestyle factors are ignored. Stress, poor nutrition, or harsh hair care can undermine even the best device. Combining technology with good self-care, a balanced diet, and possibly medication or professional treatments is more likely to yield success.

18.17 Motivation and Psychological Boost

Technology can boost motivation by making progress visible. A man might get discouraged if he does not notice results day to day. But seeing photos from three months ago side by side with current images can reveal small but real gains. This evidence often encourages continued effort.

Chapter 19: Personalized Treatment Plans

For men dealing with hair loss, no single approach works for everyone. Different factors—like genetics, hormone levels, health conditions, daily habits, and personal preferences—all combine to affect how well a certain strategy might work. That is why a personalized plan often leads to the best results. Instead of trying random products or relying on one-size-fits-all guidelines, a tailored strategy can respect a person's specific hair loss pattern, budget, and lifestyle.

In this chapter, we will walk through the key elements of forming a personalized plan. We will see how consultations, tests, and regular follow-ups can shape goals and track improvements. We will also look at how to combine different methods—medical treatments, daily routines, and mental support—to build a plan that fits well into everyday life.

19.1 The Importance of Individual Factors

19.1.1 Genetics and Family History

Some men inherit a strong genetic tendency for hair loss, while others have milder risks. Knowing whether male relatives lost hair early, or whether thinning appeared gradually, can offer clues about likely outcomes. Genetic tests, like the TrichoTest mentioned earlier, give more detailed information on how each person might respond to treatments. This insight can guide whether to try certain medications or focus on other solutions.

19.1.2 Hormone Levels

A major cause of male pattern baldness is sensitivity to dihydrotestosterone (DHT). Men with higher levels of 5-alpha reductase (the enzyme that converts testosterone to DHT) or a greater sensitivity to DHT might need therapies that block this hormone more directly (for example, finasteride or dutasteride). Checking hormone levels through blood tests can confirm if these treatments are a priority.

19.1.3 Health Conditions and Medications

Sometimes other health issues like thyroid imbalances, nutrient shortfalls, or autoimmune disorders speed up hair loss. Medications for conditions like high blood pressure or depression can also cause shedding as a side effect. A thorough health review helps ensure no underlying problem is overlooked. If an issue is found, addressing it might fix or reduce hair thinning.

19.1.4 Lifestyle and Habits

Men with high-stress jobs, poor eating patterns, or harmful habits such as smoking may see hair thinning worsen. A personalized plan often includes small shifts in everyday habits—such as improved nutrition, stress management, or better sleep. While these do not erase genetic factors, they can help hair remain stronger and more resilient.

19.2 Meeting with Specialists

19.2.1 The Role of a Dermatologist

Dermatologists specialize in skin, hair, and nails. They can diagnose the root cause of hair loss through visual exams, pull tests, or scalp biopsies if needed. A dermatologist might also run blood work to check for thyroid problems, anemia, or other conditions. After clarifying what is going on, they can suggest medications or guide a person to other solutions, such as specialized shampoos or scalp treatments.

19.2.2 Trichologists and Hair Clinics

While not medical doctors, trichologists focus on hair and scalp health. They can help with scalp hygiene, product advice, or mild conditions like flaking. For more serious hair loss, a trichologist may collaborate with a doctor or dermatologist. Some men find that seeing both a dermatologist and a trichologist covers all bases—from medical to cosmetic concerns.

19.2.3 Endocrinologists

When hormone issues are suspected, an endocrinologist can run a deeper evaluation. This may be necessary if a thyroid disorder or significant testosterone imbalance is involved. The endocrinologist can offer medication adjustments or additional tests, ensuring the hair loss plan addresses any underlying hormonal triggers.

19.2.4 Mental Health Experts

Because hair loss can affect self-esteem, men who experience deep stress or sadness might visit a counselor or therapist. In a personalized approach, managing emotional well-being is as important as dealing with the physical aspects of hair thinning. This can prevent negative thoughts from undermining the overall plan.

19.3 Combining Different Methods

A personalized plan might include several elements at once. For example:

1. **Medical Treatment:** Finasteride, minoxidil, or low-level laser therapy.
2. **Lifestyle Changes:** Better nutrition, consistent sleep, or a moderate exercise routine.
3. **Scalp Care:** Using gentler shampoos, routine scalp massage, or anti-dandruff treatments if needed.
4. **Emotional Support:** Staying active in a support group or seeing a counselor for anxiety or self-image concerns.
5. **Cosmetic Steps:** Hair fibers, a new haircut, or scalp micropigmentation to boost appearance.

The plan can be adjusted over time if certain parts are not effective or if new needs arise.

19.4 Setting Realistic Goals

19.4.1 Goals vs. Guarantees

No matter how good a plan is, hair regrowth is rarely guaranteed. The main aims often include slowing further loss, thickening areas that still have active follicles, and improving scalp health. Some men see partial regrowth, while others maintain their current coverage. Setting clear, reachable goals helps avoid disappointment and keeps expectations in check.

19.4.2 Time Frames

Treatments that are proven, such as finasteride or minoxidil, often need 3–6 months to show obvious changes. Even hair transplants can require up to a year to reveal final results. Recognizing these time frames is key. If a plan is abandoned too soon, men might miss the chance to see meaningful progress.

19.4.3 Budgeting for Hair Care

A thorough plan might include monthly medication costs, clinic visits, or specialized products. Men who want a hair transplant or scalp micropigmentation may need to save and plan for the expense. Creating a realistic budget ensures that financial stress does not sabotage the plan partway through.

19.5 Examples of Personalized Plans

To illustrate how different factors come together, consider these three hypothetical scenarios:

1. **Case A: Mild Early Thinning**
   - **Health Check:** Blood tests reveal slightly low iron levels, but no major hormone issues.
   - **Plan:** Improve nutrition with more iron-rich foods, begin minoxidil once daily, schedule monthly scalp photos, join an online support group for tips.

    - **Goal:** Slow hairline recession and add mild thickness.
2. **Case B: Moderate Hereditary Hair Loss**
    - **Health Check:** Hormone levels are normal, but there is a strong family pattern of balding.
    - **Plan:** Start finasteride to lower DHT, plus a laser cap for 15 minutes three times a week. Seek a counselor if self-image concerns are high. Possibly look into a hair transplant if the thinning progresses or if the front hairline remains a concern after one year.
    - **Goal:** Maintain current hair and possibly regrow some in the crown region.
3. **Case C: Significant Thinning with Stress**
    - **Health Check:** Mild thyroid underactivity plus high stress at work. The man also has unhealthy eating patterns.
    - **Plan:** Adjust thyroid medication with an endocrinologist. Start minoxidil for the crown area. Speak with a nutritionist for balanced meals. Practice simple stress reduction, like a 10-minute relaxation exercise each morning. Visit a dermatologist to consider scalp micropigmentation in the future.
    - **Goal:** Improve scalp environment by controlling the thyroid issue and stress, slow or minimize further thinning, and possibly get a cosmetic enhancement if the thinning remains bothersome.

These scenarios show how each plan is unique, guided by the men's distinct medical and lifestyle factors.

19.6 Tracking Progress

19.6.1 Regular Checkpoints

Many specialists recommend checkups every three to six months to see how well the plan is working. These sessions could involve scalp exams, updated photos, or blood tests if a health condition is being managed. Tracking changes step by step helps fine-tune the plan quickly instead of waiting a year to spot failures.

19.6.2 Photo Documentation

As mentioned in Chapter 18, using consistent angles and lighting can reveal subtle progress. Some men start a simple routine: taking a few pictures under the same bathroom light monthly. This helps them remain objective; the slow pace of hair growth can make changes hard to see day to day.

19.6.3 Feedback from Others

Sometimes a barber or stylist notices improvements—or new thinning patches—before the person does. Trusted family members or friends can also provide honest input if asked. However, it is crucial to ask for constructive feedback, not casual remarks that might be discouraging.

19.7 Adjusting the Plan if Needed

19.7.1 Evaluating Treatment Responses

Suppose a man used minoxidil for six months with no visible difference. A dermatologist might advise waiting another three months or considering a stronger medication or combination therapy. Or, if a man is on finasteride and experiences unwanted side effects, the plan might shift to a different approach.

19.7.2 Considering Surgical or Cosmetic Options

If medical or lifestyle steps are not enough, a man might explore a hair transplant, scalp micropigmentation, or wearing a hairpiece. In a personalized plan, these methods are not last-resort "defeats" but part of a legitimate spectrum. The timing depends on personal comfort, finances, and how advanced the thinning has become.

19.7.3 Reevaluating Emotional Factors

Sometimes the plan stalls because stress or negative self-view is not being addressed. Checking in with a mental health professional, or resuming counseling sessions, can reignite motivation to follow daily steps like applying treatments or sticking to scalp care routines.

19.8 Common Roadblocks and Solutions

1. **Lack of Consistency:** Busy schedules cause missed medication doses or laser therapy sessions.
   - **Solution:** Use calendar reminders, phone alarms, or accountability with a friend.
2. **Costs:** Prescription meds, special shampoos, or clinic visits can strain finances.
   - **Solution:** Compare generic versions or ask about payment plans. Some clinics offer package deals for repeated sessions.
3. **Impatience:** Men may expect quick changes, then quit.
   - **Solution:** Remind oneself of the hair growth cycle's slow nature. Mark diaries with milestones.
4. **Social Pressure:** Teasing or negative remarks from others can lower confidence.
   - **Solution:** Lean on supportive networks, set boundaries, or talk to a professional counselor.
5. **Information Overload:** Conflicting advice on forums or from friends can cause confusion.
   - **Solution:** Identify a primary doctor or dermatologist to weigh various options. Rely on proven information over rumors.

19.9 The Role of Self-Advocacy

A personalized plan works best when a man feels in control. Speaking up if a medication causes issues, questioning a doctor if something is unclear, and requesting alternative treatments if necessary—these are all forms of self-advocacy. The more someone engages with their own hair loss plan, the more likely they are to stick with it and adapt it effectively.

19.10 Tips for Staying Motivated

- **Visualize the End Goal:** Whether it is a fuller crown, a stable hairline, or simply less shedding, keeping the purpose in mind aids consistency.
- **Reward Small Wins:** If monthly photos show slight improvement, treat yourself to something positive (within reason) as a motivational boost.
- **Stay Flexible:** Accept that your plan might need updates as body chemistry or life circumstances shift.
- **Involve a Friend:** Sharing progress or setbacks with a buddy can make the experience less isolating.
- **Practice Self-Kindness:** Minor relapses or missed applications happen. Avoid guilt or harsh self-criticism.

19.11 Collaborative Planning with Doctors

19.11.1 Building Rapport

Working hand in hand with a doctor or dermatologist helps tailor the plan to medical realities. Ask about potential side effects, how long to wait before switching approaches, and how to measure success. A respectful, open relationship ensures that if problems arise (like side effects), there is no fear of asking for guidance.

19.11.2 Second Opinions

If a specialist's recommendations do not resonate, or if progress stalls, getting another professional's view can provide fresh insights. It might confirm that the initial approach is valid or suggest different methods that were previously overlooked.

19.12 The Psychological Benefit of a Tailored Plan

Personalization can also ease emotional stress. Instead of feeling overwhelmed by too many random solutions or conflicting tips, a man can say, "I have a plan made for my unique situation." This sense of direction counters the hopeless feeling that hair loss is unstoppable or beyond control. Each step—whether it is applying a topical product or picking a scalp-friendly shampoo—becomes part of a purposeful routine.

19.13 Monitoring and Gathering Data

19.13.1 Keeping a Hair Journal

A basic notebook or phone app can store data about daily or weekly observations: shedding patterns, stress events, new products tried, or side effects from medication. Over time, patterns might emerge—like noticing that certain foods or stressful weeks coincide with increased fall-out. Even a quick note each day can become a valuable resource.

19.13.2 Working with Technology

Chapter 18 covered devices like scalp analyzers or laser therapy. Men might integrate these into a plan, using them consistently and noting any changes. By blending objective data (like scalp images) with personal observations, a complete picture emerges.

19.14 Tailoring for Different Stages of Hair Loss

- **Early Stage:** A plan may focus on daily treatments (minoxidil), improved eating, and mild stress reduction. Men can often see good stabilization if they start early.
- **Middle Stage:** Combination therapy becomes more common: finasteride plus laser therapy, or possibly PRP injections for extra help. Emotional and cosmetic support can also ramp up.

- **Advanced Stage:** If the top is mostly bald, a transplant or micropigmentation might be the main approach, with medication to protect the donor area or slow further recession. Scalp care remains essential to preserve any remaining natural hair.

19.15 Questions to Ask Before Finalizing a Plan

1. **What is the probable cause of my hair loss?**
2. **Are there any health concerns I need to address first (like thyroid, anemia, or nutrient gaps)?**
3. **Which treatments align with my budget and time availability?**
4. **Am I ready to commit to long-term use of medication if needed?**
5. **How will we measure improvement—photos, scalp checkups, or something else?**
6. **Who can I contact if I face side effects or new questions?**

Having these questions answered increases confidence and helps avoid surprises.

19.16 Looking Ahead

Once a personalized plan is in place, the next phase is long-term maintenance and monitoring, which is crucial for holding on to any gains. Many men find that hair care remains a steady process. Even if regrowth is minimal, slowing or halting further thinning can be a big success. In the following (and final) chapter, we will talk more about sustaining results over time, dealing with relapses, and adjusting the plan as life changes happen.

Chapter 20: Long-Term Maintenance and Monitoring

Taking steps to manage hair loss is not a short-term project. Even the best plans usually require ongoing effort to sustain improvements. Hair grows in cycles that can last for several years, so changes to the scalp and follicles might happen slowly. At the same time, hormonal shifts, life stress, or health issues can arise unexpectedly, affecting the hair's condition.

In this final chapter, we will examine how to maintain progress once a plan is set. We will look at methods for regular checkups, ways to spot warning signs early, and tips on preventing or handling relapses. We will also highlight the importance of staying flexible, since life rarely stands still—jobs change, daily habits shift, and new treatments may appear on the market.

20.1 Why Maintenance Matters

20.1.1 Keeping Gains

Men who have stabilized hair loss or achieved some regrowth through medication or laser therapy might lose that progress if they stop too soon. Finasteride and minoxidil, for example, often need continuous use. Once halted, the protective effect might fade, letting hair revert to its earlier thinning pattern.

20.1.2 Monitoring for New Issues

Over years, the body changes. A health problem like chronic stress or a thyroid imbalance can show up unexpectedly, accelerating hair loss again. Regular checkups help spot such changes before they cause serious damage to the hairline or scalp.

20.1.3 Adjusting to Age and Lifestyle

As men grow older, hormone levels can shift naturally. Some may see hair thinning speed up, even if they had mild loss before. Lifestyle factors—like intense workouts, new diets, or hectic schedules—can also influence shedding. Maintenance includes adapting to these transitions.

20.2 Ongoing Treatment Schedules

20.2.1 Daily or Weekly Routines

Some regimens require daily actions: applying minoxidil foam each morning, or taking a finasteride pill at a set time. Others, like laser therapy caps, might be used a few times each week. Consistency remains critical. Skipping sessions intermittently might slow progress or undo improvements.

To stay on track, men often set alarms on their phone or integrate the routine into an existing habit (for instance, applying minoxidil right after brushing teeth).

20.2.2 Monthly or Bi-Monthly Tasks

Tasks like taking scalp photos, restocking medication, or checking in with a support buddy can happen monthly. Some men schedule them on the same date each month so they will not forget. This ensures that small problems—like running out of medication—do not spiral into major setbacks.

20.2.3 Clinic Visits

For those with a dermatologist or trichologist, visits might be scheduled every three to six months. At these appointments, professionals can see if the scalp remains healthy, if hair loss has slowed, or if changes are needed. Men who have had a hair transplant might need a follow-up at a certain interval to monitor graft survival and scar healing.

20.3 Watching for Warning Signs

20.3.1 Increased Shedding

It is normal to lose 50–100 hairs per day. But if a man notices clumps of hair in the shower or a significant jump in shedding, it could signal a relapse or a new trigger (such as medication side effects, high fever, or shifting hormones). Paying attention to these changes early allows quick action, whether that is visiting a doctor or reevaluating a routine.

20.3.2 Scalp Discomfort

New itching, burning, or redness might point to an allergic reaction, infection, or irritation from a product. Ignoring these can worsen the scalp environment, hurting follicles. Spotting scalp problems early can prevent permanent damage.

20.3.3 Product or Medication Side Effects

Men who try new supplements or medications should watch for side effects like rashes, mood changes, or sexual function issues. Not everyone experiences them, but if they do appear, contacting a health professional promptly is wise. Adjusting dosage or switching to another treatment may resolve problems while protecting hair health.

20.4 Adjusting as Needed

20.4.1 Switching Medications

Sometimes a drug stops working well after a year or two, or side effects become a problem. A dermatologist might suggest rotating to a different class of medication or adding a second therapy. For instance, if minoxidil alone is less effective over time, combining it with a low-level laser device or PRP sessions could help.

20.4.2 Fine-Tuning Lifestyle

If stress intensifies or dietary habits slip, hair might reflect that change. Regularly reassessing one's lifestyle can ensure that healthy eating, rest, and exercise remain priorities. Even men who do not see an immediate drop in hair thickness can gain from these measures, as they also support overall health.

20.4.3 Revisiting Surgical or Cosmetic Options

Men who were not ready for a hair transplant or scalp micropigmentation earlier might decide to explore those paths if thinning has progressed. On the flip side, someone who had a transplant might look into micropigmentation to further hide any leftover scarring or to add a sense of fullness.

20.5 Staying Informed About New Developments

As Chapter 13 highlighted, research in hair loss solutions continues. Over the years, better medications, more precise surgical techniques, or gene-based therapies might become available. While it is unwise to jump at every rumor, staying mildly updated through reputable medical news or dermatologist advice can help men spot real breakthroughs.

20.6 Preventing Hair Care Burnout

20.6.1 Recognizing Weariness

Applying topical treatments daily or taking pills for years can become tedious. Some men feel worn out or resentful of the routine. If this emotional fatigue sets in, they might skip sessions or quit entirely.

20.6.2 Methods to Stay Engaged

- **Simplify the Process:** Switch to easier formulations (for example, a once-daily foam instead of a twice-daily lotion) if equally effective.

- **Combine Tasks:** Pair hair care with another habit (listening to a short podcast while applying minoxidil).
- **Regular Tracking Rewards:** Seeing photo comparisons can be a morale boost, proving that the routine is doing some good.
- **Support Network:** Friends, online forums, or family can offer encouragement on tough days.

20.7 Handling Setbacks

20.7.1 Accepting Imperfection

Hair loss plans rarely go perfectly. Life events—like relocating, family responsibilities, or financial strain—can disrupt even the most carefully structured approach. Recognizing that occasional slip-ups happen helps men avoid harsh self-blame.

20.7.2 Restarting After Breaks

If a man stops minoxidil for a month and notices a surge in shedding, it is not too late to restart. While some ground might be lost, picking up the routine again can often slow or reverse that new wave of thinning. The key is to act sooner rather than waiting months or years.

20.7.3 Learning from Mistakes

If a product caused scalp irritation in the past, note that for future decisions. If a certain clinic or brand was unreliable, avoid it next time. Each misstep can shape a better plan. In that sense, setbacks can ultimately refine long-term success.

20.8 Long-Term Emotional Management

20.8.1 Evolving Perspectives

As men mature, their view of hair loss may shift. What felt devastating at 25 might be less of a crisis at 45, especially if they have found stable relationships or career achievements. Some men become more at ease with visible thinning as they age. But others might want to keep defending hair volume as long as possible. There is no right or wrong—just personal preference.

20.8.2 Regular Emotional Check-Ins

Because hair loss can link to self-esteem, it is wise to check mental well-being from time to time. If anxiety resurfaces, or if looking at old photos sparks sadness, consider talking to a counselor or a friend. Emotional care remains a continuous element of the hair loss picture.

20.8.3 Celebrating Stability or Minor Wins

When a man sees that hair has stayed roughly the same for a year, or that a small bald patch looks denser, it is a positive sign that efforts are working. Recognizing these wins can fuel ongoing motivation. They show that with patience, stable results can be maintained.

20.9 Maintenance After Surgical Procedures

20.9.1 Post-Transplant Guidelines

Men who have had a hair transplant usually follow specific instructions to ensure grafts heal well. This might include gentle washing techniques, avoiding direct sun on the scalp for a few weeks, and not picking scabs. Over the next year, follow-ups let the doctor confirm graft survival and see if any additional sessions are desired.

20.9.2 Addressing the Donor Area

In transplants, hair is taken from a "safe zone," but this zone can still be affected by dryness, scarring, or aging. Using scalp-friendly products and keeping an eye on scarring is helpful. Some men find micropigmentation beneficial to mask minor scars, letting them keep shorter hair without visible lines.

20.9.3 Future Touch-Ups

Sometimes one transplant is enough, especially if hair loss is mild. However, men with more extensive patterns might consider a second procedure years later if thinning continues in untreated areas. Maintaining or continuing medical therapy (finasteride or minoxidil) around transplanted regions can protect non-transplanted hair from receding further.

20.10 Strategies for Different Life Phases

20.10.1 Young Adults

For men in their early or mid-20s, finishing school or starting new jobs can be hectic. Minimal routines (like once-daily minoxidil) and a mild shampoo might be most realistic. Large surgical choices may be postponed until hair loss patterns become clearer.

20.10.2 Middle Age

Men in their 30s or 40s might settle into longer-term medication use (finasteride or dutasteride) if well tolerated. Stress from work or family can rise, so balancing mental health is important. If hair loss is advanced, some men opt for a transplant at this stage, hoping for a stable improvement.

20.10.3 Older Adults

By 50s or 60s, some men choose simpler approaches, such as very short haircuts or scalp micropigmentation. Others remain committed to medication. Health factors (heart issues, diabetes) or finances might shape the plan. The main point is that hair care remains personal; there is no age limit to seeking a look that feels comfortable.

20.11 Revisiting Goals Periodically

20.11.1 Shifts in Priorities

A man may start with a strong desire to restore a youthful hairline but later find that stopping further loss is enough. Or the opposite might happen: he was content for a while but decides he wants a fuller front zone. Revisiting goals every 6 to 12 months ensures that the plan matches current wishes.

20.11.2 Tracking and Reflecting

Take time to compare scalp photos from the year before, check if stress levels have changed, or see if the budget still allows certain treatments. A short reflection can clarify if adjustments are in order.

20.12 Blending Maintenance with Overall Wellness

20.12.1 Exercise and Health

Regular exercise improves circulation, hormones, and stress levels. Though it does not directly cure genetic hair loss, it fosters a better environment for hair to stay strong. Men who keep fit tend to have more stable energy levels and are better equipped to handle daily routines.

20.12.2 Sleep and Recovery

Nighttime is when the body repairs tissues, including scalp cells. Persistent lack of sleep might weaken hair growth or worsen stress. Integrating good sleep hygiene (consistent bedtimes, minimal screen light before bed) can complement any hair plan.

20.12.3 Nutritional Choices

Dietary needs evolve over time. A man who once ate plenty of protein might reduce intake as he ages, potentially affecting hair strength. Monitoring key nutrients (protein, iron, zinc, vitamins) helps keep hair from suffering due to hidden dietary gaps.

20.13 Looking Back on the Entire Process

At some point, a man may look back at when thinning first appeared, remembering initial worries and solutions tried. Realizing how far he has come—whether by sustaining hair health, feeling less anxious about it, or trying out a new style—can be empowering. This reflection can also highlight how consistent maintenance pays off in the long run.

20.14 Community and Shared Wisdom

20.14.1 Ongoing Forums

Staying active in a hair loss community can help men remain aware of new advice or fresh product lines. It also ensures a sense of camaraderie, as others share maintenance stories. If a person previously left a forum after stabilizing hair, returning for occasional updates can keep knowledge fresh and maintain ties with supportive peers.

20.14.2 Helping Newcomers

Men who have managed hair loss successfully for years can become mentors. By answering questions, posting progress pictures, or explaining how they overcame setbacks, they help new members skip common pitfalls. Contributing knowledge not only benefits others but can reaffirm one's commitment to ongoing hair health.

20.15 Planning for Unforeseen Changes

20.15.1 Life Transitions

Major transitions—such as relocating to a different climate, changing jobs, or dealing with family health concerns—can disrupt routines. Being prepared with simpler fallback strategies can keep hair care from completely dropping off the radar during turbulent times.

20.15.2 Economic Shifts

If finances get tight, men might have to scale down on expensive therapies. Chatting with a dermatologist about cheaper generic drugs or fewer in-clinic sessions can maintain some degree of continuity.

20.15.3 Health Events

Surgeries, accidents, or serious illnesses can alter the body's resources and hormone levels. After recovering, re-evaluating hair status with a professional is wise. Temporary shedding (telogen effluvium) could occur, and adjusting the plan can speed up the return to normal.

20.16 Final Thoughts on Maintenance

Hair loss management often moves from an intense focus in the early stages to a steadier approach over the years. Many men find a stable middle ground: They do not let hair loss rule their life, but they also do not neglect it entirely. They keep up a routine that feels manageable, check scalp health occasionally, and adapt if new issues come up.

The essence of maintenance is balance: consistent enough to preserve results, flexible enough to handle changing situations. Underlying everything is a recognition that hair changes over a lifetime, but so does personal perspective. Some men become more relaxed with the idea of partial thinning, while others remain determined to fight it every step of the way. Both stances are valid if they bring self-confidence and comfort.

---

www.ingramcontent.com/pod-product-compliance
Lightning Source LLC
LaVergne TN
LVHW012105070526
838202LV00056B/5636